Pain Management

Editor

CATHERINE CURTIN

HAND CLINICS

www.hand.theclinics.com

Consulting Editor
KEVIN C. CHUNG

February 2016 • Volume 32 • Number 1

ELSEVIER

1600 John F. Kennedy Boulevard • Suite 1800 • Philadelphia, Pennsylvania, 19103-2899

http://www.theclinics.com

HAND CLINICS Volume 32, Number 1
February 2016 ISSN 0749-0712, ISBN-13: 978-0-323-41690-0

Editor: Jennifer Flynn-Briggs
Developmental Editor: Kristen Helm

Hand Clinics (ISSN 0749-0712) is published quarterly by Elsevier Inc., 360 Park Avenue South, New York, NY 10010-1710. Months of publication are February, May, August, and November. Business and Editorial Offices: 1600 John F. Kennedy Blvd., Ste. 1800, Philadelphia, PA 19103-2899. Customer Service Office: 3251 Riverport Lane, Maryland Heights, MO 63043. Periodicals postage paid at New York, NY and at additional mailing offices. Subscription price is $390.00 per year (domestic individuals), $687.00 per year (domestic institutions), $100.00 per year (domestic students/residents), $445.00 per year (Canadian individuals), $799.00 per year (Canadian institutions), $530.00 per year (international individuals), $799.00 per year (international institutions), and $256.00 per year (international and Canadian students/residents). Foreign air speed delivery is included in all *Clinics* subscription prices. All prices are subject to change without notice. **POSTMASTER:** Send address changes to *Hand Clinics*, Elsevier Health Sciences Division, Subscription Customer Service, 3251 Riverport Lane, Maryland Heights, MO 63043. Customer Service (orders, claims, online, change of address): Elsevier Health Sciences Division, Subscription **Customer Service, 3251 Riverport Lane, Maryland Heights, MO 63043. Tel: 1-800-654-2452 (U.S. and Canada); 314-447-8871 (outside U.S. and Canada). Fax: 314-447-8029. E-mail: journalscustomerservice-usa@elsevier.com (for print support); journalsonlinesupport-usa@elsevier.com (for online support).**

Reprints. For copies of 100 or more of articles in this publication, please contact the Commercial Reprints Department, Elsevier Inc., 360 Park Avenue South, New York, New York 10010-1710. Tel.: 212-633-3874; Fax: 212-633-3820; E-mail: reprints@elsevier.com.

Hand Clinics is covered in *MEDLINE/PubMed (Index Medicus), Current Contents/Clinical Medicine, EMBASE/Excerpta Medica,* and *ISI/BIOMED.*

Contributors

CONSULTING EDITOR

KEVIN C. CHUNG, MD, MS
Charles B. G. de Nancrede Professor of
Surgery, Professor of Plastic Surgery and
Orthopaedic Surgery, Chief of Hand Surgery,
University of Michigan Health System,
Assistant Dean for Faculty Affairs, Associate
Director of Global REACH, University of
Michigan Medical School, Ann Arbor, Michigan

EDITOR

CATHERINE CURTIN, MD
Associate Professor, Department of Surgery,
Palo Alto VA Health System and Division of
Plastic Surgery, Stanford University, Palo Alto,
California

AUTHORS

IAN CARROLL, MD, MS
Assistant Professor of Anesthesiology and Pain
Management, Department of Anesthesiology,
Stanford University School of Medicine,
Stanford Medicine Outpatient Center,
Redwood City, California

ELENA CASTARLENAS, PhD
Unit for the Study and Treatment of
Pain – ALGOS, Universitat Rovira i Virgili;
Research Center for Behavior Assessment
(CRAMC), Department of Psychology,
Universitat Rovira i Virgili; Institut
d'Investigació Sanitària Pere Virgili, Universitat
Rovira i Virgili, Catalonia, Spain

JOHN DAVID CLARK, MD, PhD
Anesthesia Service, Veterans Affairs Palo Alto
Health Care System, Palo Alto, California;
Department of Anesthesiology, Stanford
University School of Medicine, Stanford,
California

CATHERINE CURTIN, MD
Associate Professor, Department of Surgery,
Palo Alto VA Health System and Division of
Plastic Surgery, Stanford University, Palo Alto,
California

BETH D. DARNALL, PhD
Clinical Associate Professor, Division of Pain
Medicine, Department of Anesthesiology,
Perioperative and Pain Medicine, Stanford
Systems Neuroscience and Pain Laboratory,
Stanford University School of Medicine, Palo
Alto, California

TIMOTHY DEER, MD
President, Center for Pain Relief, Charleston,
West Virginia

ARNOLD LEE DELLON, MD, PhD
Professor of Plastic Surgery, Professor of
Neurosurgery, Johns Hopkins University,
Towson, Maryland

NICHOLAS HOWLAND, MD
Division of Plastic Surgery, University of Texas
Medical Branch, Galveston, Texas

MARK P. JENSEN, PhD
Department of Rehabilitation Medicine,
Harborview Medical Center, University of
Washington, Seattle, Washington

MARIELA LOPEZ, MD
Division of Plastic Surgery, University of Texas
Medical Branch, Galveston, Texas

SEAN MACKEY, MD, PhD
Chief, Stanford Division of Pain Medicine,
Redlich Professor, Departments of
Anesthesiology, Perioperative and Pain
Medicine, Neurosciences and Neurology,
Stanford University School of Medicine, Palo
Alto, California

PORTER McROBERTS, MD
Holy Cross Hospital, Ft. Lauderdale, Florida

MARIANO E. MENENDEZ, MD
Research Fellow, Department of Orthopaedic
Surgery, Massachusetts General Hospital,
Harvard Medical School, Boston,
Massachusetts

JORDI MIRÓ, PhD
Unit for the Study and Treatment of
Pain – ALGOS, Universitat Rovira i Virgili;
Research Center for Behavior Assessment
(CRAMC), Department of Psychology,
Universitat Rovira i Virgili; Institut
d'Investigació Sanitària Pere Virgili, Universitat
Rovira i Virgili, Catalonia, Spain

JASON E. POPE, MD
President, Summit Pain Alliance, Santa Rosa,
California

DAVID PROVENZANO, MD
President, Pain Diagnostics and
Interventional Care, Sewickley,
Pennsylvania

DAVID RING, MD, PhD
Professor, Department of Orthopaedic
Surgery, Massachusetts General Hospital,
Harvard Medical School, Boston,
Massachusetts

SUSAN W. STRALKA, PT, DPT, MS
Germantown, Tennessee

MARAL TAJERIAN, MSc, PhD
Anesthesia Service, Veterans Affairs Palo Alto
Health Care System, Palo Alto, California;
Department of Anesthesiology, Stanford
University School of Medicine, Stanford,
California

ROCÍO DE LA VEGA, PhD
Unit for the Study and Treatment of
Pain – ALGOS, Universitat Rovira i Virgili;
Research Center for Behavior Assessment
(CRAMC), Department of Psychology,
Universitat Rovira i Virgili; Institut
d'Investigació Sanitària Pere Virgili,
Universitat Rovira i Virgili, Catalonia,
Spain

ANDREW Y. ZHANG, MD
Assistant Professor of Surgery, Division of
Plastic Surgery, University of Texas Medical
Branch, Galveston, Texas

Contents

Pain is a unique somatosensory perception that can dramatically affect our ability to function. It is also a necessary perception, without which we would do irreparable damage to ourselves. In this article, the authors assess the impact of pain on function of the hand. Pain can be categorized into acute pain, chronic pain, and neuropathic pain. Hand function and objective measurements of hand function are analyzed as well as the impact of different types of pain on each of these areas.

Successful management of problems related to the hands and upper extremities begins with a comprehensive assessment of the pain experience and related factors. Pain intensity is the domain most commonly assessed, and pain relief is often the primary goal of treatment. Because pain is a private and subjective experience, self-report is considered the gold standard of pain measurement. This article describes and discusses the strengths and weaknesses of the most commonly used self-report scales used to measure hand pain intensity, and gives recommendations to help clinicians select from among the various options for measuring the intensity of hand pain.

Pain is a clinical challenge to health care providers who care for hand disorders. Pathologic pain that prevents recovery leads to dissatisfaction for both patients and providers. Despite pain being common, the root cause is often difficult to diagnose. This article reviews the examination and diagnostic tools that are helpful in identifying pathologic and neuropathic pain. This article provides tools to speed recognition of these processes to allow earlier intervention and better patient outcomes.

The intensity of pain reported for a given nociception is highly variable. Variation in pain intensity is best accounted for by stress, distress, and ineffective coping strategies. Among orthopedic surgery patients, greater intake of opioids is associated with greater pain intensity and decreased satisfaction with pain control, no matter the pathophysiology or nociception. The single most effective pain reliever is self-efficacy (the sense that one can manage and that everything will be okay).

caused by a neuroma, and joint pain of neural origin. Compressed nerve should be decompressed and depending on the intraoperative findings a neurolysis also should be performed. Painful neuroma must be resected to stop the pain generator. For a painful joint, the biomechanics of that joint must first be stable before denervation.

Upper extremity neuropathic pain states greatly impact patient functionality and quality of life, despite appropriate surgical intervention. This article focuses on the advanced therapies that may improve pain care, including advanced treatment strategies that are available. The article also surveys therapies on the immediate horizon, such as spinal cord stimulation, peripheral nerve stimulation, and dorsal root ganglion spinal cord stimulation. As these therapies evolve, so too will their placement within the pain care algorithm grounded by a foundation of evidence to improve patient safety and management of patients with difficult neuropathic pain.

According to the Institute of Medicine Relieving Pain in America report and the subsequently released National Pain Strategy, pain affects more than 100 million Americans and costs more than half a trillion dollars per year. We have a greater appreciation for the complex nature of pain and realize that it can develop into a disease in itself. We must focus on prevention of chronic pain and interdisciplinary approaches, particularly for the most persistent pain problems. For precision pain medicine to be successful, health systems must be linked with biomarkers of chronic pain and its treatment.

HAND CLINICS

RELATED INTEREST

Nursing Clinics of North America, September 2014 (Vol. 49, Issue 3)
Integrating Evidence into Practice for Impact
Debra D. Mark, Marita G. Titler, and Rene'e W. Latimer, *Editors*

THE CLINICS ARE AVAILABLE ONLINE!
Access your subscription at:
www.theclinics.com

Preface
Pain Management

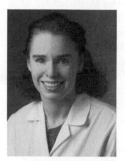

Catherine Curtin, MD
Editor

This issue of *Hand Clinics* is devoted to the subject of pain. For surgeons, pain is a common theme in patient care and can be a frustrating area of practice. Pain is a subjective experience that cannot be externally evaluated, so the health care provider has no ability to quantitatively assess the pain or its response to treatment. The subjective nature of pain can leave the provider feeling uncertain on next steps, especially when the patient complains of pain even though the tissue injury has healed. With experience, it becomes clear that refilling narcotics is not the solution for these pain patients. Yet other potential treatment options often are unfamiliar or seem to be in the domain of other disciplines. Thus, the surgeon can be stuck waiting on the availability of a pain doctor or bogged down in insurance delays before their patient gets the appropriate treatments. This issue of *Hand Clinics* does not want to make hand surgeons into pain physicians. However, the goal is to provide hand surgeons with more information and tools. Then, surgeons can ensure their patients with pain get timely and appropriate care. A hand surgeon with knowledge of the field of pain management can quickly initiate treatment and direct the patient to the most appropriate outside providers.

This overview of pain and its treatment is particularly timely as pain management is increasingly part of public discourse and heath policy goals.[1,2] Appropriate pain management is linked to quality-of-care initiatives and is a Joint Commission Standard. Pain treatment is strongly associated with patient satisfaction.[3,4] Poor pain control increases the likelihood of unplanned return to care, such as an emergency visit or readmission to the hospital. For example, we found that after distal radius fracture treatment, pain was a common cause of unplanned return to care.[5] These negative results from inadequate pain control (readmissions and decreased patient satisfaction) are now increasingly linked to financial penalties, which means that for surgeons improving pain control is not just a humanistic goal but an economic one.

Yet there are also countervailing pressures in pain management to decrease the reliance on opioids due to an epidemic of abuse of prescription medications.[6] Surgeons are caught in the middle of these forces, trying to provide adequate patient care but not contribute to inappropriate use of opioid medications. Thus, for surgeons who both cause and treat pain, it is critical to understand the many different facets of pain and its treatment.

One reason that pain care is challenging for surgeons is that most educational tools, research, and information are found outside the field of hand surgery. These other fields (mostly anesthesia) have extensively studied pain and found that a high and surprisingly consistent number of people have prolonged pain after surgery (about 20% regardless of the surgery).[7] This prolonged pain is often thought to be of neuropathic origin.[8] This *Hand Clinics* issue discusses pain with a focus on neuropathic pain and includes information from a wide array of experts from different disciplines. The issue reviews the impact of pain on hand function and looks at risk factors associated with the development of persistent pathologic pain.

This *Hand Clinics* issue presents a broad review of treatment options, including psychological, physical therapy, medication, nerve stimulation, and surgical interventions.

I hope that the information in this issue of *Hand Clinics* will provide hand surgeons with more information on familiar treatments and new strategies to use to treat their patients with pain. With a complete armamentarium, pain treatment can go from the most frustrating to a highly satisfying part of your practice. There are no patients more grateful than those you help with their pain.

Catherine Curtin, MD
Palo Alto Veterans Hospital and Stanford University
Suite 400, 770 Welch Road
Palo Alto, CA 94304, USA

E-mail address:
curtincatherine@yahoo.com

REFERENCES

1. Sifferlin A. The problem with treating pain in America. TIME. Available at: http://time.com/3663907/treating-pain-opioids-painkillers/. Accessed August 1, 2015.

2. IOM Report. Relieving pain in America. Available at: http://iprcc.nih.gov/docs/032712_mtg_presentations/IOM_Pain_Report_508comp.pdf. Accessed August 7, 2015.

3. Hanna MN, González-Fernández M, Barrett AD, et al. Does patient perception of pain control affect patient satisfaction across surgical units in a tertiary teaching hospital? Am J Med Qual 2012;27(5):411–6.

4. Maher DP, Wong W, Woo P, et al. Perioperative factors associated with HCAHPS responses of 2,758 surgical patients. Pain Med 2015;16(4):791–801.

5. Curtin CM, Hernandez-Boussard T. Readmissions after treatment of distal radius fractures. J Hand Surg Am 2014;39(10):1926–32.

6. Substance Abuse and Mental Health Services Administration. Results from the 2012 National Survey on Drug Use and Health: Summary of National Findings, NSDUH Series H-46, HHS Publication No. (SMA) 13–4795. Rockville (MD): Substance Abuse and Mental Health Services Administration; 2013.

7. Kehlet H, Jensen TS, Woolf CJ. Persistent postsurgical pain: risk factors and prevention. Lancet 2006; 367(9522):1618–25.

8. Shipton E. Post-surgical neuropathic pain. ANZ J Surg 2008;78(7):548–55.

Pain and Hand Function

Nicholas Howland, MD, Mariela Lopez, MD, Andrew Y. Zhang, MD*

KEYWORDS

- Pain • Acute pain • Chronic pain • Neuropathic pain • Hand function

KEY POINTS

- Pain is a unique somatosensory perception that can dramatically affect our ability to function.
- Pain is a necessary perception, without which we would do irreparable damage to ourselves, dramatically affecting the ability to function.
- Pain can be categorized into acute pain, chronic pain, and neuropathic pain.
- Hand function and objective measurements of hand function are analyzed as well as the impact of different types of pain on each of these areas.

INTRODUCTION

Pain is the unpleasant perception associated with actual or potential cellular damage. However, pain does not always have to be a "…useless, unjust, incomprehensible, inept abomination…" as described by J.K. Huysmans.[1] Robert Sapolsky wrote:

> Pain is useful to the extent that it motivates us to modify our behaviors in order to reduce whatever insult is causing the pain, because invariably that insult is damaging our tissues. Pain is useless and debilitating, however, when it is telling us that there is something dreadfully wrong that we can do nothing about. We must praise the fact that we have evolved a physiologic system that lets us know when our stomachs are empty. Yet at the same time we must deeply rue our evolving physiologic system that can wrack a terminal cancer patient with unrelenting pain.[2]

Pain can uniquely affect the function of the hand in a variety of ways, dependent on the type, quality, and severity of the pain. How many patients with a painful affliction of the hand have thought, *if only I didn't have this pain, I would be able to…*? And yet, one of the more intriguing aspects of pain is that without it, the impact to the hand would be just as devastating as those resulting from severe, intense pain. The necessity of pain has been thoroughly illustrated by Paul Brand, in his lifelong work with patients afflicted by leprosy. Leprosy, or Hansen disease, is caused by *Mycobacterium leprae* and can affect the peripheral nerves in patients' bodies, leading to paralysis and loss of sensation, including pain. In Brand and Yancey's book, *The Gift of Pain*, they describe their initial troubles in the postoperative care of patients with leprosy:

> Most physiotherapists in hand surgery have to coax their recuperating patients to move their fingers a little more each day…In working with leprosy patients, we fought the opposite problem of preventing them from moving their fingers too much too soon…the same hand therapist treating two identical tendon transfer recipients, one due to polio and the other to leprosy, would urge one on to greater effort, and strive to hold the other one back. Several times I had to repair tendons that had been yanked out by an overeager leprosy patient.[1]

Hand function can be significantly affected by *any* pain or *no* pain at all; thus, assessment is even more difficult. The authors describe different types of pain, which can be generally categorized

Division of Plastic Surgery, University of Texas Medical Branch, 301 University Boulevard, Galveston, TX 77550, USA
* Corresponding author.
E-mail address: dr.zhang@gmail.com

Hand Clin 32 (2016) 1–9
http://dx.doi.org/10.1016/j.hcl.2015.08.002
0749-0712/16/$ – see front matter Published by Elsevier Inc.

as acute, chronic, and neuropathic. Using specific examples of these types of pain, the authors assess how each can distinctively affect the function of the hand. The authors then describe basic hand functionality, measurements of hand function, and the complex role that pain plays in hand function.

PAIN

The mechanism of pain from stimulus to perception can be generalized into 3 stages. In the first stage of pain, the *pain signal* is the activation of pain receptors to real or perceived danger. At the second stage, the *pain message* is relayed through the central nervous system (CNS) from the spinal cord to the brain. This stage is where the gate theory of pain comes into play. The last stage is the *pain response*. After the message is relayed to higher cortical centers in the brain, a decision is made based on all incoming messages and current priorities about how to respond to the initial signal that was triggered. Pain, as a real perception, does not actually *exist* until all 3 stages have been complete.[1] Although an overly generalized description of the pain pathway, it holds true as a sound basis of understanding. Many painful diseases can be understood in terms of these 3 stages.

ACUTE PAIN

Acute pain is a physiologic response to impending or recent danger.[3] Often appearing suddenly, it is described as sharp or throbbing and may range from mild to severe. Acute pain is an essential component of the hand examination as it often helps localize and identify the causes of injury. Reproducing acute hand pain is often easy to do by observing the position of the hand, directly palpating, or performing provocative tests.

Nociception, the physiologic process of acute hand pain, involves 4 complex processes.[4] It is the rapid progression and synchronization of these processes that warn patients of injury. These processes are vital to the preservation of hand function because these serve as both alarming and protective measures.

The 4 processes of nociception include transduction, transmission, perception, and modulation.[4]

Transduction

The first process is the *pain signal.* There are free nerve endings known as nociceptors present in somatic structures, such as skin, muscles, connective tissue, bones, and joints. These nociceptors

respond to noxious stimuli, such as recent surgery; infection; bony trauma, such as fractures or dislocations; soft tissue injury, such as burns or lacerations; tendon injury; or ischemia, such as compartment syndrome. Nociceptors present on the C and A pain fibers of neurons are associated with different qualities of pain. The A fibers are larger and myelinated, making them fast conducting and primarily responsible for well-localized, sharp pain seen in acute hand pain.[4-6]

Transmission

The second stage is the *pain message.* The process begins with transmission from the nociceptors to the spinal cord and to the brain stem and thalamus.[4-6]

Perception

The third stage of pain is the *pain response.* From the brain stem and thalamus, signals are sent to cortices resulting in the perception of pain as a conscious experience. Multiple systems are activated, each accounting for different responses. For example, the reticular system results in the autonomic and motor response to pain. The somatosensory cortex interprets the intensity, quality, and location of the pain and relates it to past experiences. The limbic system is responsible for the emotional response to the pain.[4]

Modulation

After perception, pain impulses are then transmitted back through the spinal cord resulting in either increased (excitatory) or (inhibitive) impulses. Analgesia is produced by these inhibitive impulses that release opioids. This process is known as endogenous pain modulation and explains the different perceptions of pain among patients.[4-6]

CHRONIC PAIN

Chronic pain is pain lasting more than 3 month that begins as acute pain that fails to resolve. Although in many cases there is an accountable inciting event, in some there is never any known cause. Its longer presence affects patients' ability to use the hand and perform basic activities of daily living (ADL). Examining these patients is often difficult as they are apprehensive to any provocative test, palpation, or motion that may trigger an increase in pain. This pain often becomes more constant and generalized while losing the sudden, sharp, localized qualities associated with acute pain.

In contrast to acute pain, the exact physiology of chronic pain remains unclear. It is thought that after injury, several changes in the CNS occur leading to prolonged transmission and modulation of pain (with increased excitatory impulses and decreased inhibitory impulses). Some patients may develop intense or persistent pain to stimuli that are not typically associated with pain or to stimuli independent of the injury. It is in the setting of chronic pain that additional measures, including imaging, nerve tests, nerve blocks, hand therapy, and other modalities, become useful in diagnosis.

NEUROPATHIC PAIN

Neuropathic pain is produced by a primary lesion or dysfunction of the peripheral or central nervous system.[7] It can affect hand function in a very distinct manner and is described as burning or electric pain.[8] First there is nociceptive pain, which is secondary to tissue injury surrounding the involved nerves. The second component is the actual neuropathic pain during which direct injury to the nerve results in hypoesthesia (loss of touch sensitivity), hypoalgesia (decrease in localized pain), or thermal hypoesthesia (loss of cold or warm sensitivity).[9]

The molecular mechanisms underlying neuropathic pain are complex. There is research that shows that the response injury is different depending on the *type* of injury. For example, avulsion injuries involve different pathways than compression injuries or sharp rhizotomy injuries.[9] Because of these differences, neuropathic pain should be separated into lesions of the peripheral nervous system and lesions of the CNS.[10]

As pain is a complex multimodal perception, it is difficult to ascribe any particular change in hand function to a specific *type* or *cause* of pain. However, the range of effect that neuropathic pain can have on overall hand function can be illustrated with some specific examples:

Complex Regional Pain Syndrome

Patients with complex regional pain syndrome (CRPS) underscore the profound effect that pain can have on hand function. CRPS involves local pain autonomic dysfunction, atrophy, and functional impairment. A variety of trophic changes affect the hand in patients with CRPS. These changes include stiffness, edema, osteopenia, atrophy of hair/nails/skin, hypertrophy or hyperkeratosis of skin, or a combination of any of these.[7] There are 3 types of CRPS that have been described (**Table 1**). Type I has *no* identifiable peripheral nerve lesion. Type II has a diagnosed peripheral nerve lesion. Type III involves nontraumatic causes producing extremity pain.[7] The exact mechanism of CRPS is poorly understood

Table 1 Classification of CRPS	
Type 1	Reflex sympathetic dystrophy (pain, functional impairment, autonomic dysfunction, dystrophic changes without clinical peripheral nerve lesion/injury)
Type 2	Causalgia (pain, functional impairment, autonomic dysfunction, dystrophic changes with a diagnosable peripheral nerve injury)
Type 3	Other pain dysfunction problems (eg, myofascial pain)

From Jette AM. State of the art in functional status assessment. In: Rothstein JM, editor. Measurements in physical therapy, vol. 7. New York: Churchill Livingstone Inc; 1985. p. 138; with permission.

but can be described as an abnormally prolonged *normal* response to a painful stimulus.

Aside from the trophic changes and chronic pain accompanying CRPS, there is autonomic nervous system dysfunction that can lead to abnormalities in vasomotor control and thermoregulation within the extremities.

Phantom Limb Pain

Phantom limb pain (PLP) is a unique circumstance in which patients perceive painful stimuli from a previously amputated extremity. This type of pain would not seem to make a difference in function, especially given that the involved limb is *absent*; but these patients undergo significant pain that affects their ADLs as well as their ability to use their limb proximal to the amputation level.[11] PLP occurs in 54% to 85% of patients with amputation.[9] The exact mechanism of this phenomenon is unknown. There is a correlation between preamputation limb pain and postamputation phantom limb pain. Studies have also shown that epidural anesthesia or postoperative intraneural anesthesia applied to the transected nerves helps prevent the development of PLP.[12,13] This highlights the role of central sensitization in pain perception. Patients undergoing amputation may be anesthetized or unaware of the procedure, but the spinal cord is still experiencing the pain by the signals being relayed.

HAND FUNCTION

The function of the hand encompasses a broad spectrum of activities. A general classification of hand function has categorized these activities as follows[14]:

1. *Self-care*: Self-care is the ability to perform ADL, such as feeding oneself, toileting, bathing, and so forth.
2. *Occupational skills*: Occupational skills are activities requiring some higher level of training in order to maintain a livelihood within society.
3. *Perception and processing of information*: Receptors in the hand allow for the perception of pain, temperature, touch, and pressure. Other receptors send signals to the brain on position, sense, and stereognosis. The hand is one of the most densely innervated areas of the body. The somatosensory arrangement of

these inputs within the cortex, the homunculus, serves to underscore the importance of this category of hand function. (**Fig. 1**)

4. *Defense and offense*: The hand can be used itself as a weapon or tool of aggression. On the other end of the spectrum, it can be used to defend against physical attacks.
5. *Gestural expression*: The hand is able to make signals or signs to convey meaning without the need for speech.
6. *Emotive touch*: A gentle stroke of the hand, massage, or a simple caress can convey feelings of love and affection.

In relation to these categories of hand function, the digits of the hand each carry individual importance in the performance of these functions. The

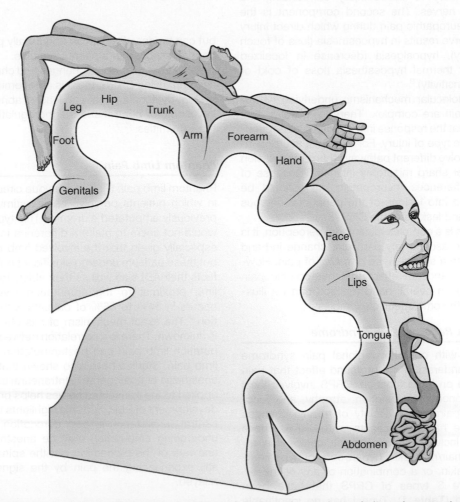

Fig. 1. The homunculus helps to illustrate the location and amount of cortical area dedicated to a particular sensation (sensory homunculus) or function (motor homunculus). The area of cortex dedicated to processing somatosensory information for a particular part of the body is not proportional to size or mass of that area; rather, it reflects the degree of innervation. The fingertips and hand display a large degree of innervation, underscoring their importance in function. (*Courtesy of* Shelby Lies, MD, Galveston, TX.)

digits have been classified into functional zones to highlight their particular roles (**Fig. 2**)[14]:

Functional zone I: The thumb, along with its metacarpal, participates in nearly all major aspects of hand function. It composes up to 40% of total hand function.[15,16]

Functional zone II: The index and middle fingers, along with their metacarpals, aid in precision grip. When paired with the thumb, these 3 digits are also known as the dynamic tripod.

Functional zone III: The ring and small fingers, along with their metacarpals, cooperate in digitopalmar holding. Contraction of the hypothenar muscles allows the small finger to move palmarly, forming a palmar cup. This movement, combined with the thumb and index finger, forms the basis of power grip.

The dynamic functions of the hand can be categorized as follows:

1. *Simple handling*: It involves simple motions of fingers, often without the need for thumb opposition (eg, static hook, dynamic hook, clamping)
2. *Precision grip/pinch grip*: It always involves the thumb, often in opposition, as well as index or other fingers to hold a small object. This maneuver is typically performed without the palm and is one of precision rather than power (eg, pulp-to-pulp pinch, tripod pinch, 5-pulp pinch, lateral pinch/key pinch). Decreased pinch and grip forces have been shown to be highly correlated with the ability to perform ADL.[17]
3. *Digitopalmar holding*: An object is placed within the palm and held with the remaining fingers, with or without the thumb (eg, position grip, power grip).
4. *Complex manipulations*: It involves higher-level cortical training that combines 2 or more of the aforementioned hand functions, often simultaneously (eg, use of chopsticks, composite grip).

It should be noted that these functions relate to the already developed, functional hand. What about the assessment of hand function in an undeveloped hand, such as a pediatric hand? Functional assessment of the pediatric hand can be challenging, and is outside the scope of this article; but a common approach to this problem is by assessing the developmental grasp observed in patients as they interact with different toys. The pediatric hand progresses through a pattern of

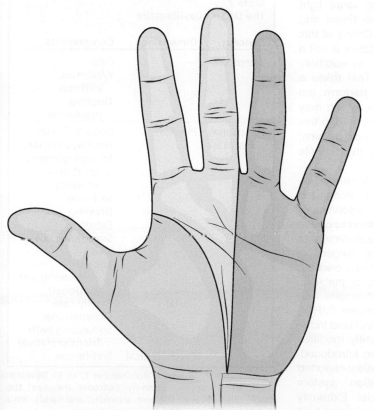

Fig. 2. The functional zones of the hand. (*Courtesy of* Shelby Lies, MD, Galveston, TX.)

grasp development from ulnar to radial and proximal to distal. This pattern has been categorized into 4 essential types of grasp: power grasp, radial digital grasp, pincer grasp, and gross grasp.[18]

MEASURING HAND FUNCTION AND PAIN

Physical function of the hand is a complex measurement that depends on multiple contexts. The evaluation of hand function is both a qualitative and quantitative process. Pain is an important factor in hand function: Hands that hurt are difficult to use. The important role of pain in hand function is clear in that several hand function measures have discrete items assessing pain. Objective tests comparing pain and hand function are lacking, as pain is an individual experience. However, several patient-reported outcome measures to assess hand function include patient reports of pain.

The ability to perform specific tasks or ADL is the most objective measure of adequate hand function.[19] In 1969, the Jebson-Taylor Hand Function Test was designed to measure the amount of time taken to complete different daily hand activities.[20] Seven subtests are completed with each hand independently. Tasks include writing, turning 3 × 5-inch index cards, picking up small common objects, simulated feeding, stacking checkers, and picking up large light and heavy objects. These tasks are timed and compared with established norms. Critics of this test suggest that time to complete tasks is not a valid predictor of hand function.[21] In addition, the Jebson-Taylor Hand Function Test takes a considerable amount of time to perform (an average of 15 minutes per subtest), which may not be feasible in a busy hand practice. Also this function measure does not include a pain domain; thus, timed tasks may not reflect the real-life impact of hand pathology.

Given a lack of validated data, the American Society for Surgery of the Hand (ASSH) recognized the need to objectively measure the outcomes of hand surgery. In 1983, the ASSH pushed to create "a universally available system for measurement of outcome of disorders treatable by surgery."[22] Since that time, several tools have been created. Classic tools include the Disabilities of the Arm, Shoulder, and Hand (DASH) questionnaire, the Michigan Hand Outcomes Questionnaire (MHQ), and Australian/Canadian Osteoarthritis Hand Index (AUSCAN), among others. More recently, modified tools and newer methods have been introduced, including the QuickDASH, the patient-reported outcomes measurement information system (PROMIS) Physical Function—Upper Extremity computer adaptive test. These methods were built primarily to increase efficiency and remove bias from questionnaires.[11] All of these measures have pain domains.

The DASH (**Table 2**) has several domains, including pain, weakness, stiffness, tingling, and numbness.[23] This tool has been a reliable measure of outcomes in a broad range of disorders, such as shoulder impingement, basal joint arthritis, and cubital tunnel syndrome.[24] The DASH is organized as a 30-item, self-reported questionnaire. There are 3 questions that specifically address pain: pain in general, pain during activity, and the effect of pain on the ability to sleep. The QuickDASH is a shorter, validated, 11-item questionnaire. It includes 2 questions specific to pain: pain in general and the effect of pain on the ability to sleep. The MHQ tests 6 domains, including overall hand function, ADL, pain, work performance, aesthetics, and patient satisfaction. One of the strengths of the MHQ is that it is based on patient-reported function and disability. The MHQ pain domain addresses pain in either hand. It begins with a general question on the presence of pain, ranging from *always* to *never*. Patients responding *never* move on to the next section. For those with any amount of pain, follow-up questions include pain

Table 2 The DASH questionnaire		
Concept	**Dimensions**	**Components**
Symptoms	—	Pain
		Weakness, stiffness
		Tingling/ numbness
Functional status	Physical	Daily activities
		House/yard chores
		Shopping/errands
		Recreational activities
		Self-care
		Dressing
		Eating
		Sexual activities
		Sleep
		Sports/ performing arts (optional)
	Social	Family care
		Occupational
		Socializing with friends/relatives
	Psychological	Self-image

From Hudak P, Amadio P, Bombardier C, et al. Development of an upper extremity outcome measure: the DASH (disabilities of the arm, shoulder, and hand). Am J Ind Med 1996;29(6):602–8; with permission.

severity, effect on sleep, effect on ADL, and effect on mood. Interestingly, the initial reliability and validity testing studies of the MHQ showed that the pain domain was the strongest independent predictor of hand function. Aesthetics was the least predictive domain. This finding has led to multiple treatment guidelines based on control of patient pain as a primary means of improving function.[22]

There have been numerous studies that confirm the early findings in the MHQ and highlight the importance of pain in the function of the hand. These studies are, admittedly, snapshots of a subset of patients with a particular disease; but the findings are consistent. In one particular study of patients with hand osteoarthritis (OA), patients were treated with topical diclofenac or a placebo gel. This study was a post hoc analysis of 2 randomized controlled trials with 783 patients. The study showed a high correlation with the pain visual analog scale (VAS) and the AUSCAN functional score (r = 0.75).[25] The pain relief also significantly correlated with improvements in stiffness and global rating of disease. This study nicely showed that treating the pain improved the hand function even though the disease (arthritis) was not modified. Even more interesting, perhaps, is that the study was a pooled analysis of *all* patients: those treated with diclofenac gel and placebo. These results would suggest that even the anticipation of pain relief can significantly affect hand function, despite no actual biomechanical improvement. Another study addressing hand OA compared 10 female patients with diagnosed hand OA and 10 demographically matched female patients without hand OA. The outcomes of the Moberg Pickup Test (MPUT) and other functional hand tests were measured. There was a strong correlation between the DASH and VAS pain scores as well as the MPUT and VAS pain scores (r = 0.73). The investigators reported: "The correlation between the DASH and VAS suggests that pain might play an important role in outcomes of upper-limb functional disability assessments; however, this conclusion should be considered with caution, since other factors such as joint stiffness may also affect hand function of the study participants."[17]

There are multiple other examples/studies that show strong correlation between subjectively reported pain and objectively measured hand function. These studies encompass a broad range of upper extremity disease as well, including OA as discussed earlier, distal radius fractures,[26] humerus fractures,[27] and carpometacarpal joint arthritis,[28] to name a few. However, care must be taken when relating pain to objective hand function. Indeed, pain control should be thought of as a separate entity in regard to hand-related

outcomes. Despite the studies cited earlier, this relationship is not always repeated and is highly complex. For example, in one recent study that measured hand function and experienced pain after a distal radius fracture, pain scores were found to increase significantly between 12 and 24 months *after* treatment. This finding would be expected to have a corollary effect on overall hand function, but the DASH score in these same patients decreased consistently from 6 weeks to 24 months after treatment. At the end of 24 months, despite persistent residual pain scores, DASH scores were within typical values and not significantly different from preinjury function.[29]

The manner in which pain affects hand function is complex. On the surface, one would assume that the presence of pain alone simply makes the physical nature of performing certain tasks difficult; therefore, function is reduced. However, there is much evidence to demonstrate that pain impacts function in a variety of ways, including patient satisfaction, recovery time from injury, and psychological well-being. Understanding the interplay between *impairment* and *disability* will help to illustrate these relationships. Impairment is defined as any loss or deviation in body function and structure. Restriction or limitation of activities resulting from that impairment is disability. Disability is a more subjective measure of the impact of impairment, usually given through patient-reported questionnaires. Some recent studies have looked at impairment and disability specifically in the upper extremity.[30,31]

One study looked at the correlation between disability as measured by DASH, MHQ, and pain intensity (VAS) with impairment as measured by the American Medical Association's (AMA) guide. There was an intermediate correlation (r = 0.38) of AMA impairment with DASH, noted to be more significant in the early postinjury period than later. There was only a small correlation, however, with MHQ (r = −0.24). In regard to pain, there was *not* a significant correlation between VAS and impairment. However, pain did correlate significantly with symptoms of depression. This correlation between pain and depression has been widely reported in other studies.[30] One group hypothesized that depression could potentially account for a large part of the variation in DASH scores for similar impairment. They attempted to control for depression in DASH scores in hopes of reducing this amount of variability. What they found was a significant reduction in variation when controlling for depression, but the reduction was only marginal.[30] They concluded that disability is complex and that controlling for a single variable could not adequately reduce variability in reported outcomes. Other studies have shown that this pain-depression relationship is secondary to a variety of factors, including different coping skills (praying and hoping), decreased self-efficacy, and other coping mechanisms (diverting attention, ignoring pain sensations, increasing activity).[31–33]

SUMMARY

Pain can have a profound effect on the function of the hand. And yet, it is also a necessary component of maintaining good hand function. The functions of the hand as described earlier can be affected by different types of pain, including acute pain, chronic pain, and neuropathic pain. When treating patients with a hand dysfunction, or any patient for that matter, one must recognize that pain is the symptom, *not* the illness.[1] Objective measurement tools of hand function can be used to demonstrate relief of pain following treatment of a particular disease. This relief, however, does not necessarily correlate with an improvement in function. The effect of pain on hand function walks a narrow line between protecting the hand against further damage, and hindering the needed function of the hand.

REFERENCES

1. Brand P, Yancey P. The gift of pain: why we hurt & what we can do about it. Grand Rapids (MI): Zondervan; 1997. p. 3–331.
2. Sapolsky R. Stress and pain. In: Why zebras don't get ulcers: the acclaimed guide to stress, stress-related diseases, and coping. 3rd edition. New York: Henry Holt and Company; 2004. p. 186–201.
3. Ko SM, Zhou M. Central plasticity and persistent pain; drug discovery today: disease models. Pain Anaesth 2004;1(2):101–6.
4. Wood S. Anatomy and physiology of pain. Nursing Times 2008. Available at: http://www.nursingtimes.net/nursing-practice/specialisms/pain-management/anatomy-and-physiology-of-pain/1860931.article.
5. Calvino B, Grilo RM. Central pain control. Joint Bone Spine 2006;73(1):10–6.
6. Farquhar-Smith P. Anatomy, physiology and pharmacology of pain. Anaesth Intensive Care Med 2007;9(1):3–7.
7. Koman LA, Poehling GG, Smith BP, et al. Complex regional pain syndrome. In: Wolfe SW, Hotchkiss RN, Pederson WC, et al, editors. Green's operative hand surgery. 6th edition. Philadelphia: Elsevier Churchill Livingstone; 2011. p. 1959–88.
8. Basbaum AI, Jessell TM. The perception of pain. In: Kandel ER, Schwartz JH, Jessell TM, editors.

9. Teixeira MJ, da Paz GS, Bina MT, et al. Neuropathic pain after brachial plexus avulsion—central and peripheral mechanisms. BMC Neurol 2015;15:73–81.
10. Treede RD, Jensen TS, Campbell JN, et al. Neuropathic pain: redefinition and a grading system for clinical and research purposes. Neurology 2008; 70(18):1630–5.
11. Doring AC, Nota S, Hageman M, et al. Measurement of upper extremity disability using the patient-reported outcomes measurement information system. J Hand Surg Am 2014;39:1160–5.
12. Bach S, Noreng MF, Tjellden NU. Phantom limb pain in amputees during the first 12 months following limb amputation, after preoperative lumbar epidural blockade. Pain 1988;33:297–301.
13. Malawer MM, Buch R, Khurana JS, et al. Postoperative infusional continuous regional analgesia: a technique for relief of postoperative pain following major extremity surgery. Clin Orthop 1991;266:227–37.
14. Yu HL, Chase RA, Strauch B. Terminology for functions and movements of the hand. In: Atlas of hand anatomy and clinical implications. St. Louis (MO): Mosby; 2004. p. 30–42.
15. Slocum DB, Pratt DR. Disability evaluation for the hand. J Bone Joint Surg Am 1946;28:491.
16. Emerson ET, Krizek TJ, Greenwald DP. Anatomy, physiology, and functional restoration of the thumb. Ann Plast Surg 1996;36:180.
17. Nunes PM, de Oliveira DG, Aruin AS, et al. Relationship between hand function and grip force control in women with hand osteoarthritis. J Rehabil Res Dev 2012;49(6):855–66.
18. Ho ES. Measuring hand function in the young child. J Hand Ther 2010;23(3):323–8.
19. Andersen KG, Christensen KB, Kehlet H, et al. The effect of pain on physical functioning after breast cancer treatment: development and validation of an assessment tool. Clin J Pain 2015;31(9):794–802.
20. Jebsen RH, Taylor N, Trieschmann RB, et al. An objective and standardized test of hand function. Arch Phys Med Rehabil 1969;50:311–9.
21. Jette AM. State of the art in functional status assessment. In: Rothstein JM, editor. Measurements in physical therapy, vol. 7. New York: Churchill Livingstone Inc; 1985. p. 137–68.
22. Chung KC, Pillsbury MS, Walters M, et al. Reliability and validity testing of the Michigan hand outcomes questionnaire. J Hand Surg Am 1998;23A(4):575–87.
23. Hudak PL, Amadio PC, Bombardier C. Development of an upper extremity outcome measure: The DASH (disabilities of the arm, shoulder and hand). The Upper Extremity Collaborative Group (UECG). Am J Ind Med 1996;29:602–8.
24. Ebersole GC, Davidge K, Damiano M, et al. Validity and responsiveness of the DASH questionnaire as

Principles of neural science. 4th edition. New York: McGraw Hill; 2000. p. 472–91.

an outcome measure following ulnar nerve transposition for cubital tunnel syndrome. Plast Reconstr Surg 2013;132(1):81e–90e.

25. Barthel HR, Peniston JH, Clark MB, et al. Correlation of pain relief with physical function in hand osteoarthritis: randomized controlled trial post hoc analysis. Arthritis Res Ther 2010;12(1):R7.

26. Swart E, Nellans K, Rosenwasser M. The effects of pain, supination, and grip strength on patient-related disability after operatively treated distal radius fractures. J Hand Surg 2012;37A:957–62.

27. Doornberg JN, van Duijn PJ, Linzel D, et al. Surgical treatment of intra-articular fractures of the distal part of the humerus: functional outcome after twelve to thirty years. J Bone Joint Surg Am 2007;89:1524–32.

28. Khan M, Waseem M, Raza A, et al. Quantitative assessment of improvement with single corticosteroid injection in thumb CMC joint osteoarthritis. Open Orthop J 2009;3:48–51.

29. Ydreborg K, Engstrand C, Steinvall I, et al. Hand function, experienced pain, and disability after distal radius fracture. Am J Occup Ther 2015; 69(1):1–7.

30. Farzad M, Asgari A, Dashab F, et al. Does disability correlate with impairment after hand injury? Clin Orthop Relat Res 2015;470(11):3470–0.

31. Calderon SA, Zurakowski D, Davis J, et al. Quantitative adjustment of the influence of depression on the disabilities of the arm, shoulder, and hand (DASH) questionnaire. Hand (N Y) 2010;5: 49–55.

32. Covic T, Adamson B, Spencer D, et al. A biopsychosocial model of pain and depression in rheumatoid arthritis: a 12-month longitudinal study. Rheumatology 2003;42:1287–94.

33. Dersh J, Polatin PB, Gatchel RJ. Chronic pain and psychopathology: research findings and theoretical considerations. Psychosom Med 2002;64: 773–86.

Self-Report Measures of Hand Pain Intensity
Current Evidence and Recommendations

Elena Castarlenas, PhD[a,b,c], Rocío de la Vega, PhD[a,b,c], Mark P. Jensen, PhD[d,*], Jordi Miró, PhD[a,b,c]

KEYWORDS

- Assessment • Pain intensity • Hand • Numerical rating scales • Visual analog scales
- Verbal rating scales • Australian/Canadian Osteoarthritis Hand Index
- Patient-Rated Wrist/Hand Evaluation

KEY POINTS

- A comprehensive evaluation of pain and its effects is an important first step in its successful management and in evaluating the effectiveness of treatments.
- Pain intensity is the most common pain domain evaluated, and self-report scales are the gold standard for its measurement.
- The use of psychometrically sound pain intensity questionnaires is fundamental to adequate assessment of pain intensity.
- Five measures (3 single-item rating scales and 2 multi-item measures) that measure pain intensity are presented and discussed: the Visual Analog Scale, the Numerical Rating Scale, the Verbal Rating Scale, the Australian Canadian Osteoarthritis Hand Index, and the Patient-Rated Wrist/Hand Evaluation.
- The strengths and weaknesses of these measures should be considered when selecting among them.

INTRODUCTION

Pain is a common complaint associated with musculoskeletal conditions, including hand-related problems.[1] Pain often has a negative impact on the quality of life of the person with pain.[2] A comprehensive evaluation of pain and its effects is an important first step in successful pain management. Pain assessment requires special attention because of the complex nature and multidimensionality of pain; a proper approach requires one to pay close attention to its sensory, emotional, affective, and cognitive aspects.[3]

Although pain is a complex biopsychosocial phenomenon influenced by many factors,[4] pain intensity is the single most common pain domain assessed in clinical settings and research studies, probably because it is the feature of pain that causes patients to seek treatment and is also the domain most commonly targeted for treatments. During the last several decades, significant gains have been made in the development and evaluation of measures that provide valid and reliable information about pain intensity. Progress in this area has allowed clinicians and researchers to

[a] Unit for the Study and Treatment of Pain – ALGOS, Universitat Rovira i Virgili, Catalonia, Carretera de Valls, s/n 43007, Spain; [b] Department of Psychology, Research Center for Behavior Assessment (CRAMC), Universitat Rovira i Virgili, Catalonia, Carretera de Valls, s/n 43007, Spain; [c] Pere Virgili Institute for Health Research (IISPV), Institut d'Investigació Sanitària Pere Virgili, Universitat Rovira i Virgili, Catalonia, Carretera de Valls, s/n 43007, Spain; [d] Department of Rehabilitation Medicine, Harborview Medical Center, University of Washington, Box 359612, 325 Ninth Avenue, Seattle, WA 98104, USA
* Corresponding author.
E-mail address: mjensen@uw.edu

Hand Clin 32 (2016) 11–19
http://dx.doi.org/10.1016/j.hcl.2015.08.010
0749-0712/16/$ – see front matter © 2016 Elsevier Inc. All rights reserved.

better understand the characteristics of the pain experience in both research subjects and patients.

Because of the private nature of pain, self-report is viewed as the gold standard for assessment. Often, patients are asked to recall pain intensity over a specified time period (eg, average pain in the past 24 hours, worst pain in the past week). Using such recall ratings has several advantages that should be considered, primary among which is that the rating comes directly from the patient, and the patient is in the best position to observe and rate his or her own pain. Furthermore, self-report rating scales, including recall rating scales, are well accepted by most patients.

One weakness of recall ratings is that they can be influenced by factors other than just pain intensity, such as emotional states (anxiety, fear), beliefs/thoughts, and other contextual factors.[5] To address these issues, clinicians and researchers should attempt to control contextual factors whenever possible; for example, by measuring pain under similar conditions such as the same time of day, in the same place, or in presence of the same people.

ASSESSING HAND PAIN INTENSITY

Pain intensity reflects the magnitude of felt pain. It is the most commonly measured pain domain, and the clinical decisions of most health practitioners are based on this parameter.[6] Patients are often familiar with the task of rating their pain intensity using self-report scales, and are usually (but not always) able to provide a reasonably rapid and valid response to rating scales. Several pain intensity scales have been developed for this purpose and have been successfully used in both clinical and research settings.

Self-report measures and rating scales of pain intensity can be used to assess the primary domain of pain intensity, or can be used as part of a questionnaire that assesses multiple pain domains. The most common single-item ratings scales used for assessing pain intensity are the Visual Analog Scale (VAS), the Numerical Rating Scale (NRS), and the Verbal Rating Scale (VRS), the strengths and weaknesses of which are presented herein and summarized in **Table 1**. The most commonly used multidimensional measures of hand function that include ratings of hand pain

intensity are the Australian/Canadian Osteoarthritis Hand Index (AUSCAN) and the Patient-Rated Wrist/Hand Evaluation (PRWHE).[a]

Single-Dimensional Pain Intensity Scales

Visual analog scales
A VAS consists of a horizontal line, usually 10 cm long, anchored by pain descriptors at each extreme; for example, "No pain" at one end and "Pain as bad as it could be" at the other end. Patients are asked to make a mark along the line to represent the point that best reflects their pain intensity. The VAS score is obtained by measuring the distance (usually in millimeters) from the "No pain" end of the line to the point that the participant has indicated. Higher scores indicate higher levels of pain. Its ease of use for many patients (except for individuals at risk for cognitive deficits such as the very elderly or persons taking high doses of analgesics that affect cognitive function) makes the VAS a well-accepted measure among many professionals and patients.

A large body of literature supports the reliability and validity of VAS scores when used in general pain populations. The VAS is also a commonly used measure in hand pain populations.[7,8] VAS scale scores have been shown to be strongly correlated with reports from other self-report scales measuring the same construct[9–11] and from observed pain behavior.[12] Discriminant validity of VAS scale scores has also been supported by research showing relatively weak associations with scores from measures of other aspects of the pain experience, such as pain unpleasantness.[13] The VAS has also been shown to be able to detect clinically important treatment effects,[14–16] including treatments of hand-related conditions.[7,17] For example, in a randomized controlled trial aimed to determine whether oxygen supplementation reduced pain associated with the use of a tourniquet in patients undergoing hand surgery, White and colleagues[17] found that the VAS was able to identify a reduction of 29% in pain scores recorded at 2-minute intervals.

In addition, the scores obtained with the VAS seem to have ratio properties[18,19]; that is, differences in pain measurement in groups (but not necessarily in individuals) represent fairly accurate estimates of differences in magnitude. For

---

[a]The Disabilities of the Arm, Shoulder, and Hand questionnaire (DASH),[82] one of the most commonly used scales in the assessment of upper extremity problems, also includes some items that assess arm, shoulder, and hand pain. However, information about the psychometric properties of this scale are not included in this article, for several reasons. First, the 30-item DASH includes only 2 that assess pain severity: one assessing overall arm, shoulder, or hand pain severity and the other pain severity when performing an activity. More importantly, the 2 pain-severity items are not scored separately into their own scale score; the DASH provides a global score of arm/shoulder/hand disability. Consequently, the DASH should not be viewed specifically as a measure of hand pain.

Table 1
Strengths and weaknesses of the single-item measures of pain intensity

Scale	Strengths	Weaknesses
Visual Analog Scale (VAS)	Easy to administer Many ("infinite") response categories Scores can be treated as ratio data Good evidence for construct validity	Some people, especially older people, have difficulty using VAS Extra step in scoring the paper-and-pencil version can take more time and adds an additional source of error
Numerical Rating Scale (NRS)	Easy to administer Many responses categories if NRS-101 is chosen Easy to score Compliance with measurement task is high Good evidence for construct validity	Limited number of response categories if the NRS-11 is used Scores cannot necessarily be treated as ratio data
Verbal Rating Scale	Easy to administer Easy to score Good evidence for construct validity Compliance with measurement task is high May approximate ratio scaling if cross-modality matching methods (or scores developed from these methods) are used	Can be difficult for persons with limited vocabulary Relatively few response categories compared with the VAS or NRS-101 If scored using the ranking method, the scores do not necessarily have ratio qualities People are forced to choose one word, even if no word on the scale adequately describes their pain intensity

Adapted from Jensen MP, Karoly P. Self-report scales and procedures for assessing pain in adults. In: Turk DC, Melzack R, editors. Handbook of pain assessment, 3rd edition. New York: Guilford Press; 2011. p. 28; with permission.

example, if the group average of VAS-measured pain intensity before treatment was 50 and 25 after treatment, we can conclude that pain intensity was reduced by half, on average. In addition, the VAS has the advantage of a very high number of response options (eg, 101 "options" if the response to a 100-mm line were measured in mm). This advantage makes the VAS theoretically better able to detect very small changes in pain, relative to scales with fewer response options, such as the Verbal Rating Scales.[20] However, it is also important to keep in mind that humans are not able to detect more than about 20 levels of sensations from "no pain" to "extreme pain." Even in the most controlled settings, many people are not able to reliably differentiate between many levels of pain.[21] Thus, measures with much fewer response categories (such as the 0–10 NRS, described later), are likely to be able to provide adequate sensitivity to change in pain intensity.

A critical weakness of the VAS is the time required to obtain the score, because the clinician has to measure the distance between the left anchor and the mark placed on the line. To address this problem, mechanical VASs have been developed. Mechanical VASs consist of a laminated piece of paper or plastic on which patients are asked to move a slider along a line to indicate their

pain level. The reverse side of the mechanical VAS provides the value associated with the distance the patient has chosen. Thus, the clinician need only look at the other side of the scale to obtain the score. Mechanical VASs have been used to assess pain intensity in general pain populations[22,23] and hand pain populations, such as in patients with carpal tunnel syndrome.[24] As with paper-and-pencil VASs, the scores from mechanical VASs have been shown to have adequate test-retest reliability[25]; they also demonstrate strong associations with the traditional paper-and-pencil VAS rating scales, and have shown an ability to detect changes in pain with treatment.[26] In addition, electronic versions of the VAS have been implemented in mobile applications,[27,28] showing good usability and acceptability as reported by the professionals who use them.

One issue to consider about is that the respondent must have a minimal level of motor skill to use a VAS. Moreover, evidence indicates that the task of converting a sensory experience (such as pain) to a line length is somewhat complex, and individuals with cognitive deficits, such as the very elderly or individuals who are recovering from recent surgery, are less able to use the VAS.[29,30] Thus, the VAS would be not recommended for use in these populations. A final problem with the

VAS is that it cannot be administered by means of an interview (eg, by telephone), which could be an important issue in conducting patient follow-up after surgery.

Numerical rating scales

The NRS is a self-report instrument that has been widely used when assessing intensity related to hand problems.[31–34] It involves asking the patient to rate his or her pain on a scale of 0 to 10 (where 0 represents "No pain" and 10 represents extreme pain, such as "Pain as bad as it could be"). Although the 0 to 10 scale is the most common form of the NRS used, if a clinician or researcher is interested in a scale with more response categories, a 0 to 20 NRS (or a 0–10 NRS whereby respondents are given the opportunity to select levels between the integers, such as "3.5" or "7.5") or even a 0 to 100 NRS may be used. However, research indicates that little, if any, improvements in reliability or validity occur when using scales with more than 11 levels,[21] suggesting that the more familiar 0 to 10 scale would be adequate in most settings. In fact, given that fewer people have difficulties using 0 to 10 scales than VAS scales, experts and consensus panels are now recommending the 0 to 10 NRS over the VAS.[35] Another advantage of NRS over the VAS is that NRSs can be administered verbally (eg, by telephone).

Another version of the NRS is the 21-point Box Scale,[36] which consists of a row of 21 boxes surrounding numbers that represent levels of pain from 0 to 100 in increments of 5, where the box labeled as 0 represents "No pain" and the one labeled as 100 represents "Pain as bad as it could be." An 11-point Box Scale has also been developed, which consists of 11 boxes representing levels of pain from 0 to 10. Patients are asked to indicate which number best represents their pain intensity by circling the box/number or placing a check mark in the box.

The NRS reports have shown excellent psychometric properties when the scale is used to measure pain intensity and, as mentioned previously, is now recommended over other measures because of its many strengths and relatively few weaknesses (eg,[35]). NRS ratings have shown positive and significant associations with those from other scales also measuring pain intensity.[10,37] NRS ratings have also shown adequate discriminant validity in relation to measures of other domains such as unpleasantness.[38] Furthermore, NRS ratings have shown good test-retest reliability and have also been demonstrated to be sensitive to treatment effects. Thus, the NRS has evidence supporting it as a responsive measure in both general pain populations (including hospital settings)[39–42] and populations with pathologic conditions of hands and upper extremities.[43,44] The NRS is easy to administer and score, which explains the high rate of compliance when NRSs are compared with other self-report measures.[45] The NRS has also been implemented in electronic devices such as smartphones,[27,46] with pain intensity ratings from such applications showing good psychometric properties even in individuals as young as 12 years.[47] A weakness of the NRS is that, in contrast with the VAS, its ratio properties have been questioned because in some samples its scores do not always have linear properties,[48,49] which limits the examiner's ability to interpret average change scores in groups of patients. However, this potential weakness does not seem to influence the reliability of its scores or its ability to detect changes in pain intensity with pain treatment.[50]

Verbal rating scale

The VRS consists of a list of words (adjectives) that describes increasing pain levels. The patient is asked to choose the single word that best describes his or her pain, and the number associated with the selected adjective is the pain intensity score for that patient. The number of words in VRSs varies widely, but 4- or 5-point VRSs are most common. In the 4-point VRS, for example, a score of 0 is given to "No pain," 1 to "Mild pain," 2 to "Moderate pain," and 3 to "Severe pain," and in the 5-point VRS an extra adjective is added, "Very severe," which is given a score of 5. VRSs have been used to measure pain intensity in hand pain conditions in several studies.[51–53]

One problem with VRSs is that they should be viewed as ordinal scales and not interval/ratio scales, because the distances between the adjectives are not necessarily equal; an increase from "mild" to "moderate" pain is not necessarily the same level of increase from "moderate" to "severe" pain, yet both represent an increase of a single point on the scale. As a result, VRSs cannot be assumed to have ratio qualities, which can complicate the interpretation of changes in pain.[54] Cross-modality matching procedures have been used to transform VRS scores into scores that have ratio properties (see Jensen and Karoly[50] for a detailed description of these procedures), but clinicians and researchers rarely use these transformations.

An important strength of VRSs is that they are easily administered and scored, especially in comparison with VASs. Of course, respondents must be familiar with the adjectives used in the measure. Importantly, despite the problems noted about

VRSs, a great deal of evidence supports their reliability and validity for detecting changes in pain with treatment. VRSs are also positively correlated with other measures of pain intensity, such as VASs and NRSs (see review by Jensen and Karoly[50]). However, research also suggests that VRSs may be less sensitive than other measures to changes in pain intensity, perhaps because of the limited response options available on the scale.[20,55,56]

Multi-Item Pain Intensity Scales

The Australian/Canadian Osteoarthritis Hand Index

The AUSCAN[57] is a self-reported 15-item scale developed to assess hand pain, stiffness, and function, whose content was developed with the involvement of health care professionals and patients.[57,58] The AUSCAN is available in more than 30 languages. Five AUSCAN items measure pain intensity, 1 item measures stiffness, and 9 items measure function. The 5 pain-related questions ask about pain associated with 5 different situations: at rest, and while gripping, lifting, turning, and squeezing objects.

In the original version of the scale, the questions refer to pain in the previous 48 hours, although the time period can potentially be varied depending on the goals of the clinician or researcher. Respondents can rate their pain intensity in response to the AUSCAN items using a 5-point Likert scale (where 0 = "No pain," 1 = "Mild pain," 2 = "Moderate pain," 3 = "Severe pain," and 4 = "Extreme pain"), a 100-mm VAS, or a 0 to 10 NRS (NRS-11).[59] It takes about 7 minutes to complete the AUSCAN items, and about 5 minutes to score the questionnaire's subscales.[60] Normative values for the AUSCAN have been published,[61] so scores can be compared with the patient's normative group.

Research supports the reliability of the AUSCAN subscale scores, with Cronbach α ranging from 0.89 to 0.98,[57,58,62–64] and test–retest reliability coefficients ranging from 0.70 to 0.86.[57,58] Construct validity of the AUSCAN pain subscale scores has been supported via strong and significant correlations with PRWHE (mentioned earlier and discussed in more detail later) pain subscale scores in a postsurgical sample.[65] Additional support for the validity of the pain subscale scores has been shown by strong and significant associations with scores from measures of other domains that should be associated with pain intensity (ie, Western Ontario & McMaster Universities Osteoarthritis Index, VAS pain, Arthritis Impact Measurement Scale 2, Short-Form 36 [SF-36]).[64]

The factor structure of the AUSCAN has also been evaluated, and research supports a 2-factor solution, with the items forming a pain intensity factor and a function factor.[62] The responsiveness of AUSCAN pain scale (both the VAS and Likert scale versions) and its comparison against the Functional Index for Hand Osteoarthritis (FIHOA; a measure of hand function)[66,67] was tested with a 6-week washout retreatment design (using a nonsteroidal anti-inflammatory drug). Standardized response means (mean difference between end of the washout and follow-ups at 1, 3, and 6 weeks) for the AUSCAN was −0.84 for the VAS version and −0.71 for the Likert scale version. The FIHOA was less sensitive to change (VAS −0.27, Likert −0.28).[58]

The AUSCAN scale was originally developed to measure pain and function in individuals with hand osteoarthritis, but it has also been validated in general community samples of individuals with and without osteoarthritis,[68] older adults with hand problems (either pain or function),[69] and in a sample that had undergone hand surgery.[65] Based on these findings, the measure seems to provide valid reports for assessing hand pain intensity in a variety of settings, including individuals recovering from hand surgery.

The original AUSCAN asks respondents to rate their usual pain (with different activities) over the past 48 hours.[57,58] There has been some variability in terms of the epoch covered, including asking about "pain in general" without a specific time range,[62,64] in the past 48 hours as in the original study,[61,68,70,71] or even in the preceding week.[69] The psychometric properties of the AUSCAN scores remain stable across all of these circumstances.

Based on these findings, if the AUSCAN were used to assess postoperative pain, the time epoch could be modified to fit the needs of the researcher. For example, the time epoch covered could be 24 hours (or even 12 hours), and the measure could be administered multiple times to track changes in pain over time. There has also been some variability in terms of the response options offered to respondents. Most studies have used the 5-point Likert scale response type,[64,65,68,70,71] although the 11-point NRS[61] and a VAS[63] have also been used as alternatives. There is no evidence to suggest that these differences in response options meaningfully alter the psychometric properties of the scale scores, so the user should consider which options fit their needs the best. For example, if the study group has limitations in cognition (older populations or patients immediately after surgery), one might prefer the easier 0 to 4 VRS to the 0 to 10 or VAS response option.

The Patient-Rated Wrist/Hand Evaluation

The PRWHE[72] is a questionnaire designed to measure pain and disability of hand, wrist, or both in daily activities, and is similar to the AUSCAN. The PRWHE evolved from the Patient-Rated Wrist Evaluation (PRWE), a questionnaire originally focused on wrist pain, which was extended to also assess hand-related conditions. The PRWHE has 15 items, 5 of which assess hand pain and 10 of which assess hand function. The pain items ask respondents to report how often they have had hand pain (1 item), the average hand pain intensity during the past week associated with 3 activities (ie, at rest, when doing a repeated movement, when lifting an object), and the worst hand pain intensity. Pain intensity is rated on an 11-point NRS from 0 ("No pain") to 10 ("The worst pain"). The items that assess function ask respondents to rate how much difficulty they had when performing specific activities that typically require use of the wrist or hand. Hand/wrist function items are rated on a scale ranging from 0 ("No difficulty in performing the activity") to 10 ("Unable to do the activity"). The final score of the pain subscale is calculated by summing the score of the 5 pain-related items, whereas the score of the function scale is computed by summing the scores of the 10 items and dividing the result by 2. A total scale score (representing a composite measure of pain and disability) can be also computed by summing the scores of both function and pain subscales. The total score can range from 0 to 100, with higher values indicating higher levels of pain and disability. In addition, the measure includes 2 optional questions about the importance of wrist/hand appearance for the patient and his or her satisfaction with hand appearance. The PRWHE is also available in Dutch,[73] Italian,[74] and Norwegian.[75]

PRWHE scores have demonstrated adequate psychometric properties when the questionnaire is used in patients presenting hand conditions. For example, the PRWHE scale scores have shown good convergent validity when correlated with reports from similar measures, such as the AUSCAN or the Disabilities of the Arm, Shoulder, and Hand (DASH) Questionnaire,[65,74] and good discriminant validity when compared with the SF-36 scale scores assessing various quality-of-life domains or the PRWHE's appearance items.[65] In addition, PRWHE scores have evidenced validity by their ability to detect changes in pain and function with treatment.[72,76–78] PRWHE scale scores have also shown adequate internal consistency and test-retest reliability.[73,74]

SUMMARY AND RECOMMENDATIONS

Pain is a subjective experience, and self-report scales are the most common (and appropriate) measures for assessing pain intensity. The 5 measures described in this article for assessing hand pain intensity have all demonstrated adequate to excellent psychometric properties, and each one has strengths and weaknesses. In selecting which measure to use (eg, a single-item scale such as the VRS, VAS, or NRS, or a multiple-item scale such as the pain subscale of the AUSCAN or PRWHE), researchers and clinicians must consider the strengths and weaknesses of each.

When the situation or setting calls for a simple single rating, for example, in most clinical situations when the health care provider wishes to monitor and track pain intensity over time, the 0 to 10 NRS asking patients to rate their current pain or average pain over an appropriate specified time period (eg, 12 hours, 24 hours, 48 hours, 1 week) should be considered. It is easier to use than the VAS for patients with compromised cognitive functioning, and evidence indicates that it provides enough response categories (11 of them) to allow patients to indicate different levels of pain intensity. In addition, because consensus groups in the pain field are recommending the 0 to 10 NRS over other measures,[35] NRS data are more likely to be comparable with other research findings and studies. The VAS should be considered only when the setting or situation calls for a measure with stronger ratio qualities, and a 4- or 5-point VRS should be considered when the population is expected to have more severe cognitive deficits (making even the 0–10 NRS challenging).

The multiple-item scales of pain intensity that are part of the AUSCAN and PRWHE appear very similar, and their scores have similar (strong) psychometric qualities. These scales should be considered when a more comprehensive measure of hand pain intensity is needed, for example, when the clinician or researcher wants to gather information regarding pain associated with specific activities. This approach may be particularly important given that pain while at rest is different (and may be influenced by different factors and/or different treatments) from pain associated with use of the hand.[79–81] At present, the authors cannot recommend the AUSCAN pain subscale over the PRWHE pain subscale or vice versa.

In short, the evidence indicates that clinicians and researchers could use the NRS, VAS, or VRS as a single measure or pain rating, or choose to use a multidimensional questionnaire such as the

AUSCAN and the PRWHE, as each of these has evidence supporting the reliability and validity of their scores. To aid clinicians and researchers in their choice, the authors make the following recommendations: (1) choose the NRS over the VAS (or VRS) in most situations if a very brief (but valid) measure is needed; (2) consider multidimensional measures if assessment burden is not a problem, given that these measures are more comprehensive and allow for the assessment of hand pain both at rest and with movement; (3) scores on the PRWHE and the AUSCAN have adequate validity and reliability properties, so both measures can be equally recommended.

REFERENCES

1. Palmer KT. Pain in the forearm, wrist and hand. Best Pract Res Clin Rheumatol 2003;17(1):113–35.
2. Li Z, Smith BP, Tuohy C, et al. Complex regional pain syndrome after hand surgery. Hand Clin 2010;26(2): 281–9.
3. Turk DC, Melzack R. The measurement of pain and the assessment of people experiencing pain. In: Turk DC, Melzack R, editors. Handbook of pain assessment. New York: Guilford Press; 2011. p. 3–16.
4. Gatchel RJ, Peng YB, Peters ML, et al. The biopsychosocial approach to chronic pain: scientific advances and future directions. Psychol Bull 2007; 133(4):581–624.
5. Keogh E, Hamid R, Hamid S, et al. Investigating the effect of anxiety sensitivity, gender and negative interpretative bias on the perception of chest pain. Pain 2004;111(1–2):209–17.
6. Ferrell BR, Eberts MT, McCaffery M, et al. Clinical decision making and pain. Cancer Nurs 1991; 14(6):289–97.
7. Rocchi L, Merolli A, Morini A, et al. A modified spica-splint in postoperative early-motion management of skier's thumb lesion: a randomized clinical trial. Eur J Phys Rehabil Med 2014;50(1):49–57.
8. Bolster M, Schipper C, Van Sterkenburg S, et al. Single interrupted sutures compared with Donati sutures after open carpal tunnel release: a prospective randomised trial. J Plast Surg Hand Surg 2013; 47(4):289–91.
9. Singer AJ, Kowalska A, Thode HC. Ability of patients to accurately recall the severity of acute painful events. Acad Emerg Med 2001;8(3):292–5.
10. Bahreini M, Jalili M, Moradi-Lakeh M. A comparison of three self-report pain scales in adults with acute pain. J Emerg Med 2015;48(1):10–8.
11. Jensen MP, Karoly P, Braver S. The measurement of clinical pain intensity: a comparison of six methods. Pain 1986;27(1):117–26.
12. Gramling SE, Elliott TR. Efficient pain assessment in clinical settings. Behav Res Ther 1992;30(1):71–3.
13. Huber A, Suman AL, Rendo CA, et al. Dimensions of "unidimensional" ratings of pain and emotions in patients with chronic musculoskeletal pain. Pain 2007; 130(3):216–24.
14. Jensen MP, Chen C, Brugger AM. Interpretation of visual analog scale ratings and change scores: a re-analysis of two clinical trials of postoperative pain. J Pain 2003;4(7):407–14.
15. Turner JA. Comparison of group progressive-relaxation training and cognitive-behavioral group therapy for chronic low back pain. J Consult Clin Psychol 1982;50(5):757–65.
16. Bird SB, Dickson EW. Clinically significant changes in pain along the visual analog scale. Ann Emerg Med 2001;38(6):639–43.
17. White N, Dobbs TD, Murphy GRF, et al. Oxygen reduces tourniquet-associated pain: a double-blind, randomized, controlled trial for application in hand surgery. Plast Reconstr Surg 2015;135(4):721e–30e.
18. Myles PS, Urquhart N. The linearity of the visual analogue scale in patients with severe acute pain. Anaesth Intensive Care 2005;33(1):54–8.
19. Price DD, McGrath PA, Rafii A, et al. The validation of visual analogue scales as ratio scale measures for chronic and experimental pain. Pain 1983; 17(1):45–56.
20. Breivik EK, Björnsson GA, Skovlund E. A comparison of pain rating scales by sampling from clinical trial data. Clin J Pain 2000;16(1):22–8.
21. Jensen MP, Turner JA, Romano JM. What is the maximum number of levels needed in pain intensity measurement? Pain 1994;58(3):387–92.
22. Petersen GL, Finnerup NB, Grosen K, et al. Expectations and positive emotional feelings accompany reductions in ongoing and evoked neuropathic pain following placebo interventions. Pain 2014;155(12): 2687–98.
23. Staud R, Vierck CJ, Robinson ME, et al. Overall fibromyalgia pain is predicted by ratings of local pain and pain-related negative affect—possible role of peripheral tissues. Rheumatology (Oxford) 2006;45(11):1409–15.
24. Bialosky JE, Bishop MD, Price DD, et al. A randomized sham-controlled trial of a neurodynamic technique in the treatment of carpal tunnel syndrome. J Orthop Sports Phys Ther 2009;39(10):709–23.
25. Gaston-Johansson F. Measurement of pain: the psychometric properties of the Pain-O-Meter, a simple, inexpensive pain assessment tool that could change health care practices. J Pain Symptom Manage 1996;12(3):172–81.
26. Choinière M, Amsel R. A visual analogue thermometer for measuring pain intensity. J Pain Symptom Manage 1996;11(5):299–311.

27. De la Vega R, Roset R, Castarlenas E, et al. Development and testing of painometer: a smartphone app to assess pain intensity. J Pain 2014;15(10):1001–7.

28. Jamison RN, Gracely RH, Raymond SA, et al. Comparative study of electronic vs. paper VAS ratings: a randomized, crossover trial using healthy volunteers. Pain 2002;99(1–2):341–7.

29. Herr KA, Garand L. Assessment and measurement of pain in older adults. Clin Geriatr Med 2001; 17(3):457–78.

30. Gabre P, Sjöquist K. Experience and assessment of pain in individuals with cognitive impairments. Spec Care Dentist 2002;22(5):174–80.

31. Pepper A, Li W, Kingery WS, et al. Changes resembling complex regional pain syndrome following surgery and immobilization. J Pain 2013;14(5):516–24.

32. Coluzzi F, Bragazzi L, Di Bussolo E, et al. Determinants of patient satisfaction in postoperative pain management following hand ambulatory day-surgery. Minerva Med 2011;102(3):177–86.

33. Schindele SF, Hensler S, Audigé L, et al. A modular surface gliding implant (CapFlex-PIP) for proximal interphalangeal joint osteoarthritis: a prospective case series. J Hand Surg Am 2015;40(2):334–40.

34. Patil S, Ramakrishnan M, Stothard J. Local anaesthesia for carpal tunnel decompression: a comparison of two techniques. J Hand Surg Br 2006;31(6):683–6.

35. Dworkin RH, Turk DC, Farrar JT, et al. Core outcome measures for chronic pain clinical trials: IMMPACT recommendations. Pain 2005;113(1–2):9–19.

36. Jensen MP, Miller L, Fisher LD. Assessment of pain during medical procedures: a comparison of three scales. Clin J Pain 1998;14(4):343–9.

37. Bijur PE, Latimer CT, Gallagher EJ. Validation of a verbally administered numerical rating scale of acute pain for use in the emergency department. Acad Emerg Med 2003;10(4):390–2.

38. Vranceanu A-M, Jupiter JB, Mudgal CS, et al. Predictors of pain intensity and disability after minor hand surgery. J Hand Surg Am 2010;35(6): 956–60.

39. Michener LA, Snyder AR, Leggin BG. Responsiveness of the numeric pain rating scale in patients with shoulder pain and the effect of surgical status. J Sport Rehabil 2011;20(1):115–28.

40. Childs JD, Piva SR, Fritz JM. Responsiveness of the numeric pain rating scale in patients with low back pain. Spine (Phila Pa 1976) 2005;30(11):1331–4.

41. Gaubitz M, Schiffer T, Holm C, et al. Efficacy and safety of nicoboxil/nonivamide ointment for the treatment of acute pain in the low back—A randomized, controlled trial. Eur J Pain 2015. [Epub ahead of print].

42. Winter S. Effectiveness of targeted home-based hip exercises in individuals with non-specific chronic or recurrent low back pain with reduced hip mobility: a randomised trial. J Back Musculoskelet Rehabil 2015. [Epub ahead of print].

43. Lampropoulou S, Nowicky AV. Evaluation of the numeric rating scale for perception of effort during isometric elbow flexion exercise. Eur J Appl Physiol 2012;112(3):1167–75.

44. Liu Y, Lao J, Gao K, et al. Functional outcome of nerve transfers for traumatic global brachial plexus avulsion. Injury 2013;44(5):655–60.

45. Hjermstad MJ, Fayers PM, Haugen DF, et al. Studies comparing numerical rating scales, verbal rating scales, and visual analogue scales for assessment of pain intensity in adults: a systematic literature review. J Pain Symptom Manage 2011;41(6):1073–93.

46. Price DD, Patel R, Robinson ME, et al. Characteristics of electronic visual analogue and numerical scales for ratings of experimental pain in healthy subjects and fibromyalgia patients. Pain 2008; 140(1):158–66.

47. Castarlenas E, Sánchez-Rodríguez E, Vega Rde L, et al. Agreement between verbal and electronic versions of the numerical rating scale (NRS-11) when used to assess pain intensity in adolescents. Clin J Pain 2015;31(3):229–34.

48. Hartrick CT, Kovan JP, Shapiro S. The numeric rating scale for clinical pain measurement: a ratio measure? Pain Pract 2003;3(4):310–6.

49. Price DD, Bush FM, Long S, et al. A comparison of pain measurement characteristics of mechanical visual analogue and simple numerical rating scales. Pain 1994;56(2):217–26.

50. Jensen MP, Karoly P. Self-report scales and procedures for assessing pain in adults. In: Turk DC, Melzack R, editors. Handbook of pain assessment. 3rd edition. New York: Guilford Press; 2011. p. 19–44.

51. Mizrak A, Gul R, Ganidagli S, et al. Dexmedetomidine premedication of outpatients under IVRA. Middle East J Anaesthesiol 2011;21(1):53–60.

52. Abdel-Ghaffar HS, Kalefa MA-A, Imbaby AS. Efficacy of ketamine as an adjunct to lidocaine in intravenous regional anesthesia. Reg Anesth Pain Med 2014;39(5):418–22.

53. Watts AC, McEachan J. The use of a fine-gauge needle to reduce pain in open carpal tunnel decompression: a randomized controlled trial. J Hand Surg Br 2005;30(6):615–7.

54. Bolton JE, Wilkinson RC. Responsiveness of pain scales: a comparison of three pain intensity measures in chiropractic patients. J Manipulative Physiol Ther 1998;21(1):1–7.

55. Chien C-W, Bagraith KS, Khan A, et al. Comparative responsiveness of verbal and numerical rating scales to measure pain intensity in patients with chronic pain. J Pain 2013;14(12):1653–62.

56. Jensen MP, Chen C, Brugger AM. Postsurgical pain outcome assessment. Pain 2002;99(1–2):101–9.

57. Bellamy N, Campbell J, Haraoui B, et al. Dimensionality and clinical importance of pain and disability in hand osteoarthritis: development of the Australian/

Canadian (AUSCAN) Osteoarthritis Hand. Osteoarthr Cartil 2002;10:855–62.

58. Bellamy N, Campbell J, Haraoui B, et al. Clinimetric properties of the AUSCAN Osteoarthritis Hand Index: an evaluation of reliability, validity and responsiveness. Osteoarthr Cartil 2002;10:863–9.

59. AUSCAN Osteoarthritis Index—AUSCAN 3.1 Hand Osteoarthritis. Available at: http://womac.com/auscan/. Accessed May 25, 2015.

60. Poole J. Measures of hand function. Arthritis Care Res (Hoboken) 2011;63(S11):S189–99.

61. Bellamy N, Wilson C, Hendrikz J. Population-based normative values for the Australian/Canadian (AUSCAN) Hand Osteoarthritis Index: part 2. Semin Arthritis Rheum 2011;41(2):149–56.

62. Allen K, Jordan J, Renner J, et al. Validity, factor structure, and clinical relevance of the AUSCAN Osteoarthritis Hand Index. Arthritis Rheum 2006; 54(2):551–6.

63. Moon K, Lee S, Kim J, et al. Cross-cultural adaptation, validation, and responsiveness of the Korean version of the AUSCAN Osteoarthritis Index. Rheumatol Int 2012;32:3551–7.

64. Slatkowsky-Christensen B, Kvien TK, Bellamy N. Performance of the Norwegian version of AUSCAN—a disease-specific measure of hand osteoarthritis. Osteoarthr Cartil 2005;13:561–7.

65. MacDermid J, Wessel J, Humphrey R, et al. Validity of self-report measures of pain and disability for persons who have undergone arthroplasty for osteoarthritis of the carpometacarpal joint of the hand. Osteoarthritis Cartilage 2007;15(5):524–30.

66. Dreiser RL, Maheu E, Guillou GB. Sensitivity to change of the functional index for hand osteoarthritis. Osteoarthritis Cartilage 2000;8(Suppl A): S25–8.

67. Dreiser RL, Maheu E, Guillou GB, et al. Validation of an algofunctional index for osteoarthritis of the hand. Rev Rhum Engl Ed 1995;62(6 Suppl 1):43S–53S.

68. Allen K, DeVellis R, Renner J, et al. Validity and factor structure of the AUSCAN Osteoarthritis Hand Index in a community-based sample. Osteoarthr Cartil 2007;15(7):830–6.

69. Dziedzic K, Thomas E, Myers H, et al. The Australian/Canadian Osteoarthritis Hand Index in a community-dwelling population of older adults: reliability and validity. Arthritis Care Res (Hoboken) 2007;57(3):423–8.

70. Haugen I, Moe R, Slatkowsky-Christensen B, et al. The AUSCAN subscales, AIMS-2 hand/finger subscale, and FIOHA were not unidimensional scales. J Clin Epidemiol 2011;64:1039–46.

71. Allen K, Jordan J, Renner J, et al. Relationship of global assessment of change to AUSCAN and pinch and grip strength among individuals with hand osteoarthritis. Osteoarthr Cartil 2006;14:1281–7.

72. MacDermid J, Tottenham V. Responsiveness of the disability of the arm, shoulder, and hand (DASH) and patient-rated wrist/hand evaluation (PRWHE) in evaluating change after hand therapy. J Hand Ther 2004;17(1):18–23.

73. Brink SM, Voskamp EG, Houpt P, et al. Psychometric properties of the patient rated wrist/hand evaluation—Dutch language version (PRWH/E-DLV). J Hand Surg Eur Vol 2009;34(4):556–7.

74. Fairplay T, Atzei A, Corradi M, et al. Cross-cultural adaptation and validation of the Italian version of the patient-rated wrist/hand evaluation questionnaire. J Hand Surg Eur Vol 2012;37(9):863–70.

75. Reigstad O, Vaksvik T, Lütken T, et al. The PRWHE form in Norwegian—assessment of hand and wrist afflictions. Tidsskr Nor Laegeforen 2013;133(20): 2125–6.

76. Packham T, MacDermid JC. Measurement properties of the patient-rated wrist and hand evaluation: Rasch analysis of responses from a traumatic hand injury population. J Hand Ther 2013;26(3): 216–23.

77. Vermeulen GM, Brink SM, Slijper H, et al. Trapeziometacarpal arthrodesis or trapeziectomy with ligament reconstruction in primary trapeziometacarpal osteoarthritis: a randomized controlled trial. J Bone Joint Surg Am 2014;96(9):726–33.

78. Prosser R, Hancock MJ, Nicholson LL, et al. Prognosis and prognostic factors for patients with persistent wrist pain who proceed to wrist arthroscopy. J Hand Ther 2012;25(3):264–9.

79. Hansen TB, Stilling M. Equally good fixation of cemented and uncemented cups in total trapeziometacarpal joint prostheses. A randomized clinical RSA study with 2-year follow-up. Acta Orthop 2013; 84(1):98–105.

80. Sagerfors M, Gupta A, Brus O, et al. Patient related functional outcome after total wrist arthroplasty: a single center study of 206 cases. Hand Surg 2015; 20(1):81–7.

81. Skott H. Palmar shelf arthroplasty for rheumatoid wrist arthritis: long-term follow-up. Am J Orthop (Belle Mead NJ) 2014;43(7):316–20.

82. Hudak PL, Amadio PC, Bombardier C. Development of an upper extremity outcome measure: the DASH (disabilities of the arm, shoulder and hand). The Upper Extremity Collaborative Group (UECG). Am J Ind Med 1996;29(6):602–8.

Pain Examination and Diagnosis

Catherine Curtin, MD

KEYWORDS

- Pain • Complex regional pain syndrome • Neuropathic pain • Neuroma • Examination • Diagnosis

KEY POINTS

- Pain that is persistent is often of neuropathic origin.
- Patient descriptors of their pain can suggest pain of a neuropathic quality.
- Careful examination can help localize nerves that are pain generators.
- Diagnostic blocks are a critical step to confirming the location of pain generators.

INTRODUCTION

Pain management is an important component of the treatment of hand disorders. Pain limits patients' abilities to participate in therapy and can ruin a technically perfect procedure. Recognizing when pain has moved beyond the expected healthy response to a pathologic process allows clinicians to aggressively treat pain as its own separate disorder. This persistent pain is often neuropathic in origin and thus may require different treatment approaches.[1] This article reviews physical examination and additional diagnostic tests to identify when pain is pathologic and where likely pain generators reside.

First it is necessary to review some pain-related terminology.

Musculoskeletal Pain

Musculoskeletal pain is pain generated from injured tissue. Patients complain of a throb, ache, tenderness to palpation, which is often the expected pain after injury.

Neuropathic Pain

Neuropathic pain is defined by the International Association for the Study of Pain (IASP) as "pain caused by a lesion or disease of the somatosensory nervous system."[2]

Neuropathic pain is the focus of this issue because this is the pain that can persist long after the tissue has healed.

Allodynia

Allodynia is pain caused by a stimulus that does not normally provoke pain.[2] This type is the pain that occurs when the skin is lightly touched.

Dysesthesia

According to the IASP Web site, dysesthesia is "an unpleasant abnormal sensation, whether spontaneous or evoked."

Complex Regional Pain Syndrome

Complex regional pain syndrome (CRPS) is a chronic pain condition with pain out of proportion to the injury, and shows skin or vasomotor changes in the affected extremity.[3] This is a clinical diagnosis and patients must have pain out of proportion to the injury. They must also report at least 1 symptom in 3 of the 4 categories shown in **Box 1**.

This work was supported by an RR&D pilot grant RX000487 from the US Department of Veterans Affairs Rehabilitation and Research and Development Service.
Disclaimer: The contents of this work do not represent the views of the US Department of Veterans Affairs or the United States government.
Department of Surgery, Palo Alto VA Health System, 770 Welch Road, Suite 400, Palo Alto, CA 94304, USA
E-mail address: curtincatherine@yahoo.com

Hand Clin 32 (2016) 21–26
http://dx.doi.org/10.1016/j.hcl.2015.08.006
0749-0712/16/$ – see front matter Published by Elsevier Inc.

Box 1
Diagnostic criteria for CRPS

Must report at least 1 symptom in 3 of the following categories:

1. Sensory: hyperalgesia and/or allodynia

2. Vasomotor: temperature asymmetry, and/or skin color changes, and/or skin asymmetry

3. Sudomotor/edema: edema, and/or sweating changes, and/or sweating asymmetry

4. Motor/trophic: decreased range of motion, and/or motor dysfunction (weakness, tremor, dystonia), and/or trophic changes (hair, nail, skin)

Must show at least 1 sign[a] at time of evaluation in at least 2 of the following categories:

1. Sensory: evidence of hyperalgesia (to pinprick), and/or allodynia (to light touch, and/or deep somatic pressure, and/or joint movement)

2. Vasomotor: evidence of temperature asymmetry and/or skin color changes, and/or asymmetry

3. Sudomotor/edema: evidence of edema, and/or sweating changes, and/or sweating asymmetry

4. Motor/trophic: evidence of decreased range of motion, and/or motor dysfunction (weakness, tremor, dystonia), and/or trophic changes (hair, nail, skin)

[a] A sign is counted only if it is observed at the time of diagnosis.
From Harden RN, Oaklander AL, Burton AW, et al. Complex regional pain syndrome: practical diagnostic and treatment guidelines, 4th edition. Pain Med 2013;14(2):184; with permission.

HISTORY

The history is the first step to understanding the pain process and can alert the clinician to the possibility of a neuropathic pain component that is separate from the soft tissue injury.

Pain Quality

The descriptors of pain that patients provide can be very informative. Neuropathic pain is often described as a shooting or burning pain. Patients complain of dysesthesias. They may describe their pain as the skin feeling like it is raw, bugs are crawling on it, or a vice sensation. These types of descriptions should alert providers to the potential of a neuropathic pain generator.

Pain Severity

Pain that is more severe than is explained by the trauma should be a red flag that the patient is at risk for prolonged pain (this is true both preoperatively and postoperatively). Severe preoperative pain is one of the strongest risk factors for transitioning to chronic pain.[4]

Pain Duration

Duration of pain is an important clue to whether pain is becoming a maladaptive process. If pain is a healthy protective response, it should ease and eventually resolve when the tissue injury has healed. Pain that continues after the tissue has healed becomes a disorder of its own. Multiple studies of postsurgical pain have found that about 20% of patients have persistent postsurgical pain.[5] However, when does the transition to persistent pain happen? The time to pain resolution likely varies depending on the severity of the inciting trauma. We studied minor hand surgeries (open carpal tunnel release and trigger release) to try to understand the pain trajectory after minor hand surgery. After surgery, the patients were called daily to ask whether they still had surgical pain (**Fig. 1**). Median time to pain resolution was 16 days. Patients who still had pain after 1 month had different pain trajectories, with high risk of pain continuing for weeks or months. For hand surgeons, the message from this study was that, for minor hand surgery, if a patient still has pain 1 month after a procedure, then the patient is entering the pathologic pain category; these are the patients who require increased pain-reducing interventions: therapy, medications, and so forth.

Pain Catastrophizing

This is a psychological maladaptive behavior to pain. Research is increasingly showing the importance of pain catastrophizing as a risk for prolonged pain and poor recovery after trauma. There are measures for this, including the Pain Catastrophizing Scale, but these may be difficult to implement in a busy clinical practice.[6] Patient statements such as "I feel this pain is going to ruin my life" or "I don't think I can go on with this pain" should alert the provider that pain catastrophizing may be a component affecting the patient's recovery. If the patient seems to be ruminating on the pain or having catastrophic thoughts in relation to the pain, the clinician should consider the possibility of a psychological behavior that is contributing to the pain experience.

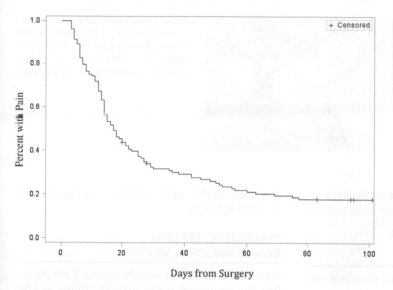

Fig. 1. Pain trajectory after open carpal tunnel and trigger finger release.

Percent with Pain

Days from Surgery

PHYSICAL EXAMINATION

The physical examination has 2 roles. It can help confirm whether the pain seems to be neuropathic in origin, and it can help identify pain-generating sites.

Inspection

First the examiner notes the patient's general distress. The provider should be concerned about pain as its own separate pathologic process if the patient is extraordinarily uncomfortable, apprehensive, and holding the hand in the injured-arm posture (adducted at shoulder, elbow flexed, hand supinated).

Most hand surgeons are aware of some of the physical signs of CRPS, such as edema, shiny skin, and temperature changes (**Fig. 2**). These

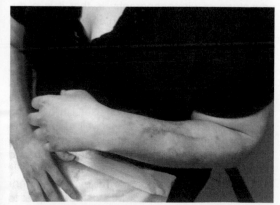

Fig. 2. Left arm of a patient with CRPS after melanoma excision.

signs can also be seen in patients with neuropathic pain who do not have enough of the clinical signs to merit a diagnosis of CRPS. However, the presence of these sudomotor changes is a clue to a neuropathic pain component.

Some patients after surgery have pain localized in the scar. The scar can be tender to light touch or palpation. On inspection, examiners often notice that, at the area of most pain, the scar is depressed or slightly widened (**Fig. 3**). These signs point to a injured cutaneous nerve in the scar.

Motor

Subtle changes in motor can alert clinicians to areas of nerve entrapment. (The caveat is that, if the patient is in severe pain, the motor examination has limited value.) The motor examination advocated by Hagert and colleagues[7] is a useful tool to understand potential nerve entrapments that could generate pain. The key to this examination is to evaluate both arms simultaneously or alternate specific muscle tests between the arms. (In contrast with the more traditional method of recording all of 1 arm's motor examination and then following sequentially with the other arm.) By examining the muscle groups bilaterally, the examiner is able to see subtle differences in strength between the limbs that would otherwise be missed. Subtle areas of weakness can point to areas of nerve compression and potential pain generators.

Palpation

Allodynia, or pain to light touch, is a clue to a neuropathic pain process. If the skin is lightly

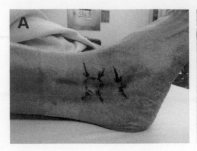 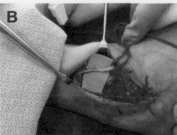

Fig. 3. (*A*) Painful scar of the ankle; note the area of depression at the point of most pain (*B*). During surgery the neuroma was found directly below the depressed scar.

touched and it is painful or unpleasant, then the pain is not originating from a deeper musculoskeletal problem.

Cold Perception

Changes in perception of temperature are well known in patients with neuropathy and neuropathic pain. There are calibrated systems to test patients' perceptions of pain (quantitative sensory testing),[8] including thermal changes. For busy clinicians, a quick and inexpensive way to assess these changes is to use ice. A piece of ice is put in a finger of an examination glove. The ice is placed on the arm in the same area on the affected and normal side. The patient is asked to assess whether the coldness is the same on both sides. Cutaneous areas with differences in cold perception can help identify areas of nerve entrapment or injury.

Tinel Sign

The Tinel sign is a well-known tool in the hand surgeon's skill set. The Tinel sign can help point to areas of nerve compression. However, this test has low sensitivity/specificity and wide variability between providers.[9,10]

Scratch Collapse Test

This test has become increasingly useful to identify nerve entrapments.[11,12] For this technique, patients are seated with upper arms at their sides and elbows at 90° flexion. The patient is asked to resist as the examiner pushes medially on a forearm (loading shoulder external rotation). The examiner then lightly scratches the skin directly over the area of the suspected nerve entrapment. Then the examiner immediately repeats the loading of the shoulder external rotation. If the patient's external rotation is weaker and collapses, this is a positive test. I find this test particularly useful for less common proximal nerve entrapments such as radial tunnel, pronator syndrome, and thoracic outlet. The scratch collapse test is

one more tool to help providers localize an area of nerve irritation.

DIAGNOSTIC TESTING
Nerve Conduction Studies

Nerve conduction is the gold standard diagnostic test for peripheral nerve injuries. These studies can identify areas of nerve compression that are contributing to pain.[13] It is essential to recognize these areas of entrapments because these entrapments are a treatable problem for the pain. However, it is important to recognize that a negative nerve conduction study does not rule out entrapment. For example, radial tunnel syndrome rarely has findings on nerve conduction studies. Also, nerve conduction studies are more challenging for more proximal nerve entrapments, where it is harder to localize areas of conduction slowing.

Ultrasonography

Ultrasonography technology is continuing to improve and there is much interest in its role in identifying peripheral nerve injuries and entrapments. There have been many studies quantifying median nerve in carpal tunnel syndrome as evaluated by ultrasonography.[14,15] An experienced ultrasonographer with state-of-the-art equipment can also assess other nerves for swelling. The advantage of ultrasonography is that it is a dynamic test and the patient can correlate the scan with the location of the pain.

MRI

MRI also has improving technology, which has expanded its utility in diagnosis of peripheral nerve injury. MRI neurogram has been useful in localizing lesions of peripheral nerves as well as providing information about the surrounding anatomy.[16] On T2-weighted images with saturation increased signal can identify the area of the nerve lesion.[17,18] Although at this point its role for more distal entrapments remains limited, MRI can be helpful to identify more proximal nerve entrapments such as cubital tunnel and thoracic outlet (**Fig. 4**).

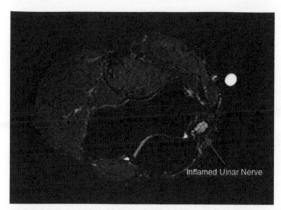

Inflamed Ulnar Nerve

Fig. 4. MRI of the ulnar nerve at the elbow. Note the bright ulnar nerve, which is so swollen that individual fascicles can be identified.

Diagnostic Blocks

Diagnostic blocks with local anesthetic are an invaluable tool for localizing and then guiding the treatment of neuropathic pain. Patients often cannot localize their pain, which makes anatomically focused treatment challenging. Blocking suspected nerves proximally can greatly assist in the understanding and treatment of the pain. We work with our pain colleagues who use ultrasonography to identify the nerve and place the blocks. There are 2 key steps to using diagnostic blocks. First, if the surgeon is not doing the block, the person administering the block must understand that the block must be localized to treating 1 nerve at a time (a field block of the forearm that resolves the pain is not useful). Second, the patient must understand the test. The important time to assess the block is during the first hour after administration of the local anesthetic. At that time the patient needs to perform the activities that aggravate the pain and assess how much of the pain was relieved. If you do not explain that the first hour is the time you are interested in, the patient may say that the block did not work because the pain returned after the local anesthetic wore off. Blocks are repeated on multiple nerves until the clinicians understand which nerves are the pain generators.

The second useful diagnostic block is a small amount of local placed just under the painful scar. If the local anesthetic relieves the pain, then the provider knows this is likely a scar neuroma and not a deeper pain generator (the local anesthetic should be of a small volume and superficial).

CLINICAL VIGNETTE OF A PATIENT WITH COMMON NEUROPATHIC PAIN

A patient complains of wrist pain after open reduction for distal radius fracture using a volar plate. She comes to you for a second opinion because her surgeon recommended hardware removal. She complains of burning pain on her volar wrist. She states that her radial fingers feel fat and numb. Physical examination shows a patient who is very apprehensive about the examination. She has pain with light touch on the volar forearm and decreased sensation to cold on the lateral forearm and volar thumb pad. She has several positive provocative tests: Tinel and scratch collapse over the carpal tunnel as well as a positive carpal compression. The affected hand is slightly more swollen. Radiograph shows a healed fracture with slightly long proximal screw. Nerve conduction study shows slowing of the median nerve across the wrist. Diagnostic blocks of the median nerve proximal to the palmar cutaneous nerve provide 25% relief. Block of the lateral antebrachial cutaneous provides 75% relief. Treatment is directed toward treating both the carpal tunnel syndrome and injury to the lateral antebrachial cutaneous nerve.

SUMMARY

Pain complaints are often an area of great frustration and confusion for providers of hand care. Understanding the division between healthy soft tissue pain and pathologic neuropathic pain is an important first step, and allows a course correction in the treatment plan. If a neuropathic component is suspected then careful history, examination, and diagnostic testing can help pinpoint the pain generator. Once you know where and what is generating the pain, then appropriate treatment can be initiated.

REFERENCES

1. Shipton E. Post-surgical neuropathic pain. ANZ J Surg 2008;78(7):548–55.
2. IASP taxonomy. Available at: http://www.iasp-pain.org/Taxonomy#Peripheralneuropathicpain. Accessed June 22, 2015.
3. Harden R, Bruehl S. Diagnostic criteria: the statistical derivation of the four criterion factors. In: Wilson PR, Stanton-Hicks M, Harden RN, editors. CRPS: current diagnosis and therapy. Seattle (WA): IASP Press; 2005. p. 45–58.
4. Kalkman CJ, Visser K, Moen J, et al. Preoperative prediction of severe postoperative pain. Pain 2003; 105(3):415–23.

5. Kehlet H, Jensen TS, Woolf CJ. Persistent postsurgical pain: risk factors and prevention. Lancet 2006;367(9522):1618–25.

6. Sullivan MJ, Bishop SR, Pivik J. The Pain Catastrophizing Scale: development and validation psychological assessment. Psychol Assess 1995;7(4): 524–32.

7. Hagert CG, Hagert E, Slutsky DJ. Manual muscle testing: a clinical examination technique for diagnosing focal neuropathies in the upper extremity. Upper extremity nerve repair: tips and techniques. A Master Skills publication. Rosemont (IL): American Society for Surgery of the Hand; 2008. p. 451–66.

8. Shy ME, Frohman EM, So YT, et al. Quantitative sensory testing: report of the Therapeutics and Technology Assessment Subcommittee of the American Academy of Neurology. Neurology 2003;60(6): 898–904.

9. Heller L, Ring H, Costeff H, et al. Evaluation of Tinel's and Phalen's signs in diagnosis of the carpal tunnel syndrome. Eur Neurol 1986;25(1):40–2.

10. Lifchez SD, Means KR Jr, Dunn RE, et al. Intra- and inter-examiner variability in performing Tinel's test. J Hand Surg Am 2010;35(2):212–6.

11. Cheng CJ, Mackinnon-Patterson B, Beck JL, et al. Scratch collapse test for evaluation of carpal and cubital tunnel syndrome. J Hand Surg Am 2008;33(9): 1518–24.

12. Blok RD, Becker SJ, Ring DC. Diagnosis of carpal tunnel syndrome: interobserver reliability of the blinded scratch-collapse test. J Hand Microsurg 2014;6(1):5–7.

13. Koh SM, Moate F, Grinsell D. Co-existing carpal tunnel syndrome in complex regional pain syndrome after hand trauma. J Hand Surg Eur Vol 2010;35(3): 228–31.

14. Buchberger W, Schön G, Strasser K, et al. High-resolution ultrasonography of the carpal tunnel. J Ultrasound Med 1991;10:531–7.

15. Abrishamchi F, Zaki B, Basiri K, et al. A comparison of the ultrasonographic median nerve cross-sectional area at the wrist and the wrist-to-forearm ratio in carpal tunnel syndrome. J Res Med Sci 2014;19(12): 1113–7.

16. Kollmer J, Bendszus M, Pham M. MR neurography: diagnostic imaging in the PNS. Clin Neuroradiol 2015. [Epub ahead of print].

17. Bendszus M, Wessig C, Solymosi L, et al. MRI of peripheral nerve degeneration and regeneration: correlation with electrophysiology and histology. Exp Neurol 2004;188(1):171–7.

18. Cudlip SA, Howe FA, Griffiths JR, et al. Magnetic resonance neurography of peripheral nerve following experimental crush injury, and correlation with functional deficit. J Neurosurg 2002;96(4): 755–9.

Factors Associated with Greater Pain Intensity

Mariano E. Menendez, MD, David Ring, MD, PhD*

KEYWORDS

• Pain intensity • Nociception • Pathophysiology • Impairment • Illness • Magnitude of disability

KEY POINTS

- The intensity of pain reported for a given nociception is highly variable.
- Variation in pain intensity is best accounted for by stress, distress, and ineffective coping strategies.
- Among orthopedic surgery patients, greater intake of opioids is associated with greater pain intensity and decreased satisfaction with pain control, irrespective of pathophysiology or nociception.
- The single most effective pain reliever is self-efficacy (the sense that one can manage and that everything will be alright).

INTRODUCTION

Nociception is the physiology of actual or potential tissue damage. Pain is the cognitive, emotional, and behavioral response to nociception. Pain intensity for a given nociception varies substantially depending on mindset and circumstances (stress, distress, and coping strategies).

Pinch the back of your hand. Notice the pain. Stop pinching and the pain dissipates. Pinching creates changes in the hand that signal potential tissue damage (nociception). Pinching the back of your hand does not hurt that much. But if an ant at a picnic bit the back of your hand and you noticed that you had put your hand down by an ant hole and there were several ants crawling on your hand, that might hurt more. If you had an ant phobia—myrmecophobia—or an allergy to ant bites, you would be frightened and that bite might be extremely painful.

The most common symptoms patients bring to a hand surgeon are pain and numbness. We surgeons spend our days meeting patients in pain and hearing their stories. Even the most junior hand surgeons are aware of the substantial variation in pain for a given nociception. Consider trigger finger: some patients can snap a severe trigger finger repeatedly and report no pain, whereas others find it difficult to demonstrate even a single triggering event.

Hand surgeons are biased to believe that there is a pathophysiologic explanation for the differences in pain intensity; that there is some biochemical, molecular, or biomechanical explanation for the variations in pain intensity. Experts have labeled this frame of reference the biomedical model of illness.[1] In the biomedical model, every illness (the state of being unwell) can be reduced entirely to its underlying disease (pathophysiology), in other words, to a malfunctioning in the human machinery.

But humans are not machines. We think, we interpret, and we have emotions. The evidence is clear that a better model for human illness behavior is the biopsychosocial model.[2] The biopsychosocial model emphasizes that illness is owing to a combination of disease (bio), mindset (psycho), and circumstances (social).[2] The biopsychosocial framework explains variations in pain intensity.[3,4]

Disclosure Statement: The authors certify that they had nothing of value related to this study.
Department of Orthopaedic Surgery, Massachusetts General Hospital, Harvard Medical School, 55 Fruit Street, Yawkey Center, Suite 2100, Boston, MA 02114, USA
* Corresponding author.
E-mail address: dring@partners.org

VARIATION IN PAIN INTENSITY FOR A GIVEN NOCICEPTION

It is easier to understand the subjective aspects of illness such as pain intensity and magnitude of disability now that we can quantify them. When the Disabilities of the Arm, Shoulder, and Hand (DASH) questionnaire[5] was introduced, we started having all our patients complete it. We observed that the range of DASH scores for a given diagnosis was remarkable, despite a relatively narrow range of severity in pathophysiology. After all, no matter how bad a trigger finger or trapeziometacarpal (TMC) arthrosis get, they still involve just 1 joint of 1 digit. But patients with a single trigger digit can rate themselves anywhere from zero symptoms or disability (a mere curiosity) to a score of 80 out of 100, indicating near complete and intensely painful incapacity (**Fig. 1**).[6]

The TMC joint is 1 spot where everyone eventually gets arthritis (**Fig. 2**).[7,8] Take a moment to consider what this means. It means that most of the patients in a hand surgeon's office aged 60 and older have TMC arthrosis. However, only a fraction of those patients are seeking help with pain at the TMC joint. Most of them have adapted to the TMC arthrosis and do not consider it a problem.[9]

MINDSET AND CIRCUMSTANCES

The lack of correlation between pathophysiology/impairment and symptom intensity and magnitude of disability is curious. As the curious become inquisitive, the most useful insights come from experts outside of our discipline: psychologists and sociologists, the experts of the workings of the human mind and the experts on human social relationships and institutions.

Every hand surgeon understands secondary gain. A perplexing discrepancy between disease and illness with a correspondingly limited response to treatment are the hallmark of a person who benefits from being ill (usually by gaining advantage in some form of dispute, but sometimes just for the attention of loved ones). Patients who derive secondary gain from illness are not typically feigning illness (malingering). Secondary gain is an example of the unconscious effect of circumstances on symptoms and disability.

Hand surgeon trepidation in treating patients involved in a dispute indicates our ability to recognize and adapt to the psychosocial aspects of illness. But it is also an example of an important pitfall: the tendency to categorize patients (eg, "comp" or "non-comp," "crazy or sane"). This natural human cognitive bias has its advantages in situations of high consequences, where snap judgments could determine life or limb. But it gets us into trouble when we are treating patients.

The influence of circumstances (eg, culture or secondary gain) and mindset (eg, stress, distress, or maladaptive responses to symptoms) is not an all-or-none phenomenon. It is not "are you depressed?" but rather "how depressed are you today?" Categorizing emphasizes the false mind–body dichotomy and reinforces the stigma associated with psychological and sociologic aspects of illness: "you are broken," or "you don't measure up." Anticipating, measuring, and treating human illness behavior on its continuum is more accurate and will make screening and treatment more appealing to patients and surgeons. When distress and effective coping strategies are evaluated on

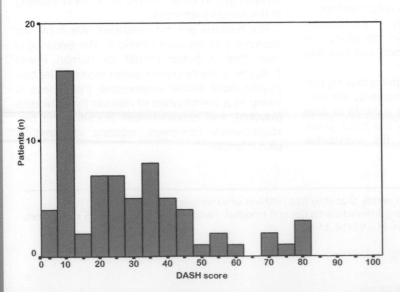

Fig. 1. Histogram of the distribution of Disabilities of the Arm, Shoulder, and Hand (DASH) scores in patients with a trigger finger. (*From* Ring D, Guss D, Malhotra L, et al. Idiopathic arm pain. J Bone Joint Surg Am 2004;86–A(7):1389; with permission.)

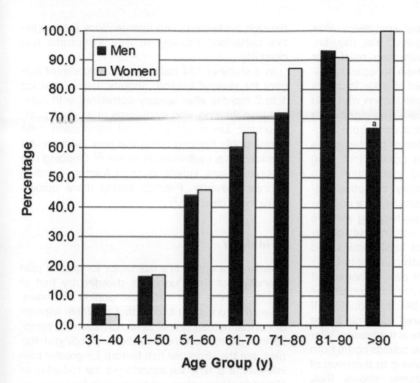

Fig. 2. The prevalence of trapeziometacarpal arthrosis increases with age in both men and women. [a] There were only 6 men older than 90 years in the study cohort; the prevalence among men in this age group is not reliable. (*From* Becker SJ, Briet JP, Hageman MG, et al. Death, taxes, and trapeziometacarpal arthrosis. Clin Orthop Relat Res 2013;471(12):3741; with permission.)

the continuum on which they are experienced, the conclusions amounts to common sense: the more confidence, adaptiveness, and resiliency, the better one's health.[10]

We talk about the "straight shooters" and we think we can pick them out. But do not forget that sociopaths (eg, Munchausen syndrome) can be quite charming. Humility is an important quality for a hand surgeon. Remember: to err is human. Expect to misjudge patients to some degree some of the time.

Extensive study in several disciplines has identified the risk factors for greater pain intensity for a given pathophysiology and nociception: stress, distress, and ineffective coping strategies. The effects of external strife (divorce, illness, financial problems, job insecurity)[11–14] and internal strife (depression and anxiety)[15–17] on symptom intensity and magnitude of disability amount to common sense. When our tank is low, we are not as adaptive and resilient. The influence of maladaptive coping strategies is less intuitive.[18–20]

The normal human response to symptoms (pain in particular) is to feel protective (avoid harm, allow healing) and prepare for the worst ("if I don't get rid of this symptom, I won't be able to..."; "this will only get worse"). This primordial human tendency (catastrophic thinking) helps us to limit damage from hot, sharp, or heavy objects, but is off the mark for the vast majority of daily pains. We can turn this "safety system" off or at least filter it when we work out, play sports, recover from an injury, or adapt to a chronic problem. The sense that everything will be all right and that we can achieve our goals is called self-efficacy. These normal human instincts are the factors that best account for the wide variation in symptoms and disability for a given pathophysiology.[18,20]

THE LIMITS OF BIOMEDICAL TREATMENT

Minor elective hand surgery (eg, for trigger finger, carpal tunnel syndrome) creates a relatively narrow and consistent nociceptive stimulus, but a wide variation in postoperative pain intensity and disability.[4] The gap between objective pathophysiology and disability and pain intensity after minor hand surgery is mediated strongly by psychosocial factors.[4] In a cohort of 120 patients undergoing minor hand surgery, maladaptive coping strategies and symptoms of depression were the strongest correlates of magnitude of disability and pain intensity at suture removal. This is also true for nonoperative procedures such as corticosteroid injection for trigger finger: catastrophic thinking and symptoms of depression correlated with pain during and the day after the injection.[21]

The limits of a biomedical-centered philosophy are highlighted by response to treatment. Most patients in countries other than the United States and

Canada take little or no opioid analgesics after musculoskeletal injury or surgery.[22] Yet, they are comfortable and satisfied with pain relief. For instance, Dutch patients who take nonopioid analgesics after operative treatment of ankle fractures report less pain and greater satisfaction with pain relief compared with Americans managed with opioids.[23] Among patients recovering from fracture surgery in the United States, greater intake of opioids is associated with greater (not less) pain intensity and decreased satisfaction with pain control, irrespective of injury, operative procedure, or surgeon.[24–27] Analogously, in a population of opioid-naïve patients undergoing elective total joint arthroplasty, greater pain intensity correlated with intake of more (not less) opioids and with decreased satisfaction with pain control.[28]

The opioid-centric model of pain management was promoted by pharmaceutical companies and advocates (many with ties to industry). It contributed to the current opioid epidemic in the United States. Opioid overdose is the leading killer of young adults and most of the opioids come from physicians, either directly or owing to diversion of excess opioids.[29] The evidence shows that, among patients with orthopedic injury and surgery, greater opioid use is actually a risk factor for greater pain intensity and a marker of greater psychological distress. An emphasis on greater opioid use for nonmalignant pain created an epidemic that can only be solved by addressing the risk factors for greater pain intensity.

PEACE OF MIND IS THE BEST PAIN RELIEVER

The evidence is consistent and compelling: the single most effective pain reliever for a given pathophysiology is peace of mind. The more we respond to nociception with catastrophic thinking, the more we are in pain and the less we can do. On the contrary, the more we feel secure and self-assured in response to nociception (self-efficacy), the less pain we experience and the more we can accomplish. Indeed, it seems that when Dutch patients break their ankle and have surgery they think, "This is going to hurt," whereas many Americans wonder, "Why am I hurting?"

Maladaptive coping strategies are consistently identified as predominant drivers of the wide variation in symptoms and disability.[18,20,26] Excessive catastrophic thinking and low self-efficacy are not only strongly linked to greater musculoskeletal pain intensity and disability,[18,20,26,30] but are also associated with ongoing use of opioid analgesics after both elective and nonelective orthopedic surgery.[27] It seems worthwhile to promptly recognize and address these ineffective coping strategies

through evidence-based interventions (eg, cognitive behavioral therapy) to limit symptoms and disability.

In a study of 154 patients who underwent surgery for skeletal trauma, ongoing use of opioids 1 to 2 months after surgery correlated with catastrophic thinking, and symptoms of anxiety, posttraumatic stress disorder, and depression, with catastrophic thinking being the only independent predictor in a multivariable model.[27] Ongoing use of opioids was independent of fracture location or injury severity. Patients taking more opioids were more disabled.[27]

SUMMARY

Greater nociception is a risk factor for greater pain intensity, but its influence is dwarfed by that of stress, distress, and ineffective coping strategies. Given the consistent finding that treatable aspects of normal human illness behavior, such as symptoms of depression and less effective coping strategies, are the strongest risk factors for greater pain intensity, it is time we abandoned the reductionist biomedical and opioid-centric models for pain management and embraced the biopsychosocial model, incorporating the effective techniques of cognitive–behavioral therapy and its variations.

REFERENCES

1. Wade DT, Halligan PW. Do biomedical models of illness make for good healthcare systems? BMJ 2004;329(7479):1398–401.
2. Engel GL. The need for a new medical model: a challenge for biomedicine. Science 1977; 196(4286):129–36.
3. Henderson M, Kidd BL, Pearson RM, et al. Chronic upper limb pain: an exploration of the biopsychosocial model. J Rheumatol 2005;32(1):118–22.
4. Vranceanu AM, Jupiter JB, Mudgal CS, et al. Predictors of pain intensity and disability after minor hand surgery. J Hand Surg Am 2010;35(6):956–60.
5. Hudak PL, Amadio PC, Bombardier C. Development of an upper extremity outcome measure: the DASH (disabilities of the arm, shoulder and hand) [corrected]. The Upper Extremity Collaborative Group (UECG). Am J Ind Med 1996;29(6):602–8.
6. Ring D, Guss D, Malhotra L, et al. Idiopathic arm pain. J Bone Joint Surg Am 2004;86-A(7):1387–91.
7. Becker SJ, Briet JP, Hageman MG, et al. Death, taxes, and trapeziometacarpal arthrosis. Clin Orthop Relat Res 2013;471(12):3738–44.
8. Sodha S, Ring D, Zurakowski D, et al. Prevalence of osteoarthrosis of the trapeziometacarpal joint. J Bone Joint Surg Am 2005;87(12):2614–8.

9. Becker SJ, Makarawung DJ, Spit SA, et al. Disability in patients with trapeziometacarpal joint arthrosis: incidental versus presenting diagnosis. J Hand Surg Am 2014;39(10):2009–15.e8.

10. Ring DC. CORR Insights(R): What is the role of mental health in primary total knee arthroplasty? Clin Orthop Relat Res 2016;173(1):164–5.

11. Brekke M, Hjortdahl P, Kvien TK. Severity of musculoskeletal pain: relations to socioeconomic inequality. Soc Sci Med 2002;54(2):221–8.

12. Jablonska B, Soares JJ, Sundin O. Pain among women: associations with socio-economic and work conditions. Eur J Pain 2006;10(5):435–47.

13. Katz WA. Musculoskeletal pain and its socioeconomic implications. Clin Rheumatol 2002;21(Suppl 1):S2–4.

14. Urwin M, Symmons D, Allison T, et al. Estimating the burden of musculoskeletal disorders in the community: the comparative prevalence of symptoms at different anatomical sites, and the relation to social deprivation. Ann Rheum Dis 1998;57(11):649–55.

15. Cotchett MP, Whittaker G, Erbas B. Psychological variables associated with foot function and foot pain in patients with plantar heel pain. Clin Rheumatol 2015;34(5):957–64.

16. Ring D, Kadzielski J, Fabian L, et al. Self-reported upper extremity health status correlates with depression. J Bone Joint Surg Am 2006;88(9):1983–8.

17. Isatali M, Papaliagkas V, Damigos D, et al. Depression and anxiety levels increase chronic musculoskeletal pain in patients with Alzheimer's disease. Curr Alzheimer Res 2014;11(6):574–9.

18. Bot AG, Doornberg JN, Lindenhovius AL, et al. Long-term outcomes of fractures of both bones of the forearm. J Bone Joint Surg Am 2011;93(6):527–32.

19. Menendez ME, Bot AG, Hageman MG, et al. Computerized adaptive testing of psychological factors: relation to upper-extremity disability. J Bone Joint Surg Am 2013;95(20):e149.

20. Teunis T, Bot AG, Thornton ER, et al. Catastrophic thinking is associated with finger stiffness after distal radius fracture surgery. J Orthop Trauma 2015. [Epub ahead of print].

21. Julka A, Vranceanu AM, Shah AS, et al. Predictors of pain during and the day after corticosteroid injection for idiopathic trigger finger. J Hand Surg Am 2012;37(2):237–42.

22. Lindenhovius AL, Helmerhorst GI, Schnellen AC, et al. Differences in prescription of narcotic pain medication after operative treatment of hip and ankle fractures in the United States and The Netherlands. J Trauma 2009;67(1):160–4.

23. Helmerhorst GT, Lindenhovius AL, Vrahas M, et al. Satisfaction with pain relief after operative treatment of an ankle fracture. Injury 2012;43(11):1958–61.

24. Bot AG, Bekkers S, Arnstein PM, et al. Opioid use after fracture surgery correlates with pain intensity and satisfaction with pain relief. Clin Orthop Relat Res 2014;472(8):2542–9.

25. Nota SP, Spit SA, Voskuyl T, et al. Opioid use, satisfaction, and pain intensity after orthopedic surgery. Psychosomatics 2014;56:479–85.

26. Vranceanu AM, Bachoura A, Weening A, et al. Psychological factors predict disability and pain intensity after skeletal trauma. J Bone Joint Surg Am 2014;96(3):e20.

27. Helmerhorst GT, Vranceanu AM, Vrahas M, et al. Risk factors for continued opioid use one to two months after surgery for musculoskeletal trauma. J Bone Joint Surg Am 2014;96(6):495–9.

28. Schumacher CS, Menendez ME, Freiberg AA, et al. Age, Tobacco Use, and Emotional Health Predict Perioperative Opioid Consumption after Total Joint Arthroplasty. Abstract submitted to the American Academy of Orthopaedic Surgeons (AAOS) Annual Meeting, 2016.

29. Inciardi JA, Surratt HL, Cicero TJ, et al. Prescription opioid abuse and diversion in an urban community: the results of an ultrarapid assessment. Pain Med 2009;10(3):537–48.

30. Bot AG, Bekkers S, Herndon JH, et al. Determinants of disability after proximal interphalangeal joint sprain or dislocation. Psychosomatics 2014;55(6):595–601.

Pain Psychology and Pain Catastrophizing in the Perioperative Setting
A Review of Impacts, Interventions, and Unmet Needs

Beth D. Darnall, PhD

KEYWORDS

- Pain psychology • Psychological • Outcomes • Catastrophizing • Perioperative • Surgical
- Surgery

KEY POINTS

- Psychological factors, including pain-related psychological factors, have a significant influence on surgical outcomes.
- Pain catastrophizing (psychological responses to actual or anticipated pain) predicts postsurgical pain intensity, opioid use, function, and the persistence of pain.
- A convergence of evidence suggests that treating pain catastrophizing and pain-related anxiety before surgery may improve recovery from surgery.
- Research on perioperative psychological interventions is sparse and limited by methodological issues, including significant variation in the timing and content of the interventions.
- Recommendations for future research include presurgical delivery of interventions (psychological prehabilitation), and standardization of outcomes to include metrics of recovery and postsurgical medication use.

INTRODUCTION

Surgical outcomes are known to be influenced by the medical complexity of the patient. An accumulation of evidence similarly shows that psychological factors affect postsurgical outcomes, thus setting the stage for the integration of psychology into models of care. Within the context of psychology, pain-specific psychological factors have emerged as particularly powerful determinants of postsurgical outcomes, at times surpassing medical characteristics or surgical variables in their predictive value. In the perioperative setting, pain is a highly salient stimulus, and psychological reactions to pain directly influence the patient experience and patients' responses to medical treatment. Accordingly, in an era of patient-centered care that focuses on cost containment and optimizing outcomes, there has been a surge of interest in the psychology of surgical patients, with a particular focus on pain psychology.

This article provides a brief overview of the literature on perioperative pain psychology in terms of relevant factors and treatments. Where possible, the content emphasizes hand surgery or hand trauma populations, although this literature is

Conflicts of interest: The author discloses no financial conflicts of interest.
Division of Pain Medicine, Department of Anesthesiology, Perioperative and Pain Medicine, Stanford Systems Neuroscience and Pain Laboratory, Stanford University School of Medicine, 1070 Arastradero, Suite 200, MC 5596, Palo Alto, CA 94304-1336, USA
E-mail address: bdarnall@stanford.edu

Hand Clin 32 (2016) 33–39
http://dx.doi.org/10.1016/j.hcl.2015.08.005
0749-0712/16/$ – see front matter © 2016 Elsevier Inc. All rights reserved.

notably limited, as well as the relevant musculo-skeletal surgery literature. In addition, gaps in understanding and patient care are identified and discussed.

In the perioperative setting, the most studied psychological factors related to pain include pain-related anxiety, general anxiety, depression, post-traumatic stress disorder, and pain catastrophizing. Although all of these psychological factors are known to correlate with pain, pain-related anxiety and pain catastrophizing are distinctly specific to the experience of pain. Pain catastrophizing is a negative mental set brought to bear in the context of actual or anticipated pain.[1] Pain catastrophizing is typically measured with the catastrophizing subscale of the Coping Skills Questionnaire[2] or with the 13-item Pain Catastrophizing Scale.[3] The Pain Catastrophizing Scale contains 3 subscales: magnification of pain, rumination of pain, or feelings of helpless about pain. Catastrophizing is a form of pain-specific psychological distress and it powerfully predicts outcomes for pain, including chronic pain intensity,[4] postsurgical pain intensity,[5–7] disability,[4] poor response to opioids,[8] greater use of perioperative opioids,[5] misuse of opioids,[9] persistent use of opioids 2 months after surgery,[10] and persistent postsurgical pain at 4-month follow-up.[11] In outpatient chronic pain samples, research suggests that pain catastrophizing has greater predictive value for treatment outcomes than disease characteristics, pain intensity, or various medical interventions.[9,12–14] A vast and varied literature has described pain catastrophizing in outpatient chronic pain. However, the number of studies that have investigated pain catastrophizing in the perioperative context remains small.

PAIN-RELATED PSYCHOLOGICAL FACTORS AND MUSCULOSKELETAL SURGERY OUTCOMES

Two systematic reviews have examined pain-related psychological predictors and correlates for chronic postsurgical pain. The first was a meta-analysis of 29 studies that examined preoperative anxiety and pain catastrophizing in patients with a postsurgical follow-up between 3 and 12 months (N = 6628).[15] Eighteen of the studies (N = 4963) involved musculoskeletal surgery, 1 of which involved shoulder surgery,[16] and none involved hand surgery. The investigators of the review noted the typical limitations of cross-study comparison with variability of constructs measured and instruments used. The types of anxiety assessed across studies varied and included state and trait anxiety, kinesiophobia (fear of movement), fear of pain, and

pain-related anxiety. In general, kinesiophobia was not a significant predictor of chronic postsurgical pain. However, the investigators reported at least moderate evidence that preoperative anxiety and pain catastrophizing were associated with the development of postsurgical chronic pain. Pain catastrophizing emerged as the strongest predictor of chronic postsurgical pain, with a maximum pooled effect size of 2.37 based on 15 studies that included 5046 patients.

> A meta-analysis of 15 studies and 5046 patients having musculoskeletal surgery revealed that presurgical pain catastrophizing was the strongest predictor of postsurgical chronic pain.[15]

The effect of psychological factors on likelihood for postsurgical chronic pain was greater in musculoskeletal surgeries compared with other surgery types (67% vs 36%, respectively). The investigators speculated that this might be caused by greater incidence of presurgical chronic pain (a known risk factor for postsurgical chronic pain) in the musculoskeletal surgery population. Most studies reported a direct association between psychological factors and chronic postsurgical pain, and no studies found reverse associations. Although results were not uniform (45% of studies found no association with psychological factors and surgical outcome) musculoskeletal surgery studies reported greater positive associations.

A systematic review examined psychological factors affecting outcomes in total hip and knee arthroplasty, the most studied surgeries with regard to pain.[17] The review included prospective studies with a minimum 6-week postsurgical follow-up. The final analysis was conducted on 35 studies, and pain catastrophizing was the only pain-specific psychological construct assessed. The investigators concluded that low preoperative mental health and pain catastrophizing negatively affected surgical outcomes. In particular, the strongest evidence was found for the direct relationship between pain catastrophizing and postsurgical pain in total knee arthroplasty. Only 1 study quantified the association with an odds ratio (OR). In that study, controlling for confounding factors, patients with greater preoperative pain catastrophizing had greater likelihood for poor outcome (OR = 2.67; 95% confidence interval, 1.2, 6.1). The outcome was defined as chronic postsurgical pain, operationalized as less than

50% improvement on the pain subscale of the Western Ontario and McMaster Universities Arthritis Index (WOMAC)[18] at 6-month follow-up.[19]

Two perioperative studies are specifically discussed below because their recency precluded inclusion in the previously mentioned systematic reviews.

In the first study, researchers examined psychological factors following musculoskeletal trauma and fracture in 152 patients.[20] Of all the factors assessed, pain catastrophizing best accounted for the variance in pain intensity and disability after skeletal trauma, controlling for depression and pain-related anxiety (measured with the Pain Anxiety Symptom Scale-20).[21] Although pain catastrophizing was the strongest overall predictor of musculoskeletal trauma outcomes, pain-related anxiety was also a significant predictor of disability in the early recovery phase (1–2 months after trauma). The same study sample was used for a separate study that examined risk factors for persistent opioid use 1 to 2 months after musculoskeletal surgery.[10] Pain catastrophizing was revealed to best predict reported persistent opioid use. Using logistic regression modeling and controlling for the injury, the surgical procedure, and the surgeon, the investigators reported that pain catastrophizing accounted for 23% of the variance in prolonged opioid use after surgery.

> Prolonged opioid use after musculoskeletal surgery (time to opioid cessation) is predicted by presurgical pain catastrophizing.

HAND SURGERY

Although the literature remains limited for hand surgery, accumulating evidence supports the impact of pain psychology in hand surgery outcomes, and in general findings align well with those from the total knee arthroplasty meta-analyses described earlier. In a recent study, researchers investigated surgical recovery in 116 patients who underwent open reduction and internal fixation for a distal radius fracture.[22] This prospective cohort study examined whether demographic variables, injury characteristics, or psychological variables were related to distance to palmar crease (finger stiffness) at suture removal and 6 weeks after surgery. Multiple variables, including pain catastrophizing, were associated with increased distance to palmar crease at suture removal. However, at 6-week postsurgical follow-up, pain catastrophizing was the only

variable associated with increased distance to palmar crease, thus pointing to delayed surgical recovery as indexed by finger motion.

In another recent prospective study, Roh and colleagues[23] conducted a prospective study on 121 patients undergoing surgery for distal radius fracture. At 4 weeks after surgery, preoperative pain-related anxiety and pain catastrophizing were significantly associated with worse outcomes: decreased wrist range of motion and grip strength. Furthermore, the association for pain-related anxiety and delayed recovery persisted at 3 months but was no longer significant at 6-month follow-up. These findings were similar to knee surgery, and suggest that early recovery after hand surgery is significantly affected by pain-related anxiety and pain catastrophizing. The investigators concluded that postsurgical outcomes may be improved by assessing and treating these factors in high-risk patients early in the recovery process. Perhaps additional benefit may be derived from brief presurgical psychological treatment because it may assist patients in decreasing anticipatory anxiety related to the surgical procedure. Furthermore, brief psychological treatment delivered 1 to 2 weeks before surgery theoretically allows patients sufficient time to encode relevant information and acquire familiarity and basic proficiency with the cognition, emotion, and physiologic regulation skills.

> Pain psychology prehabilitation that focuses on skills acquisition may improve patients' ability to control their perioperative experience, and possibly their postsurgical outcomes.

Several factors merit consideration with surgical candidates. First, many patients have pain before surgery, possibly even chronic pain. Patients also have individual, established patterns of responses to pain that include pain beliefs, cognitions, emotions and behaviors. For instance, in patients with hand fractures, catastrophizing predicted current pain, and pain-related anxiety predicted task-related pain even after controlling for injury-related variables.[24] Given that pain is an important consideration in surgical treatment, it is possible that pain catastrophizing speeds the path to surgery while simultaneously undermining surgical response. Other work has shown that postsurgical acute pain is predicted by psychological factors, including anxiety,[7] depression, and pain catastrophizing.[7] In short, pain-related psychological factors (ie, how patients respond to their pain) are predictive for pain outcomes across the continuum of injury and care.

Most of the literature attempts to distinguish patients who improve after surgery from those who do not. Less studied are the predictors for the patients who get worse after musculoskeletal surgery. One prospective study examined predictors of chronic postsurgical pain in 50 adolescents undergoing spine surgery.[25] The investigators found that, 6 months after surgery, 22% of the sample showed pain intensity that was equal to or worse than their baseline presurgical pain intensities, and that these poor surgical results were predicted by presurgical anxiety and low pain self-efficacy (catastrophizing was not measured). The findings highlight the importance of addressing psychological factors such as anxiety to attempt to mitigate chronic postsurgical pain.

Pain self-efficacy–confidence in one's ability to carry out activities even when in pain – was recently studied by Vranceanu and colleagues in 120 patients undergoing 1 of 3 types of minor hand surgery: carpal tunnel syndrome, trigger finger, or benign tumor resection.[26] The researchers found a significant correlation between postsurgical pain intensity with pain catastrophizing, pain anxiety, and pain self-efficacy. Multivariate analyses revealed that, after controlling for all factors, depression emerged as the sole significant predictor of function,[26] as indexed by scores on the Disabilities of the Arm, Shoulder, and Hand (DASH).[27] A few points merit consideration regarding the disparate findings from these 2 studies. First, the 2 studies utilized surgical samples that are divergent in location and medical complexity (spine surgery vs minor hand surgery). The considerable shared variance. Additional methodological considerations include the considerable shared variance among the psychosocial variables investigated, as well as different outcomes variables. Collectively, these studies illustrate the importance of sample characteristics and variability in study designs, all of which must be considered when interpreting findings and comparing study results.

PRACTICAL IMPLICATIONS AND TREATMENTS

In aggregate, the evidence suggests that psychological factors contribute substantially to surgical outcomes. A logical question is whether the variables can be modified to improve outcomes. The psychological component to treating pain includes an array of approaches to improve cognition and emotion regulation. Such approaches include mindfulness-based stress reduction, cognitive-behavior therapy, acceptance and commitment therapy, meditation, pain education, relaxation, hypnosis, or some combination of these approaches. In the outpatient setting, treatment typically involves 8 to 12 treatment sessions that are delivered individually or in group settings (classes). As such, typical psychobehavioral treatment of pain may involve significant patient burdens in terms of time and costs, and patients may benefit from the development of effective treatments that are brief, scalable, and broadly accessible.

The Veterans Affairs provides immediately available online tools that include the Breathe2Relax mobile application, which is a stress management and diaphragmatic breathing tool (http://t2health.dcoe.mil/mediakit/breath2relax-mobile-application). Patients who are seeking to either reduce their need for opioid medication or to simply bolster pain psychology skills may find Less Pain, Fewer Pills to be a helpful print resource, and the American Chronic Pain Association offers a wealth of helpful information on chronic pain and how to optimize self-management strategies. (http://www.acpa.org/).[28] In addition, relaxation audio files or audio CDs are a low-cost resource for patients, and are particularly useful if used daily. Relaxation audio CDs or audio files are widely available and some are created specifically for pain management and people with medical concerns.[29]

PRESURGICAL PSYCHOBEHAVIORAL INTERVENTIONS

Although the theoretic and clinical bases for presurgical psychological screening and intervention seem sound, the data from studies of the effects of presurgical mind-body therapies on postoperative outcomes are mixed.[30] A recent systematic review of 20 prospective randomized controlled trials involving presurgery and postsurgery study design (1297 patients) included studies on relaxation alone (N = 8), guided imagery combined with relaxation (N = 8), and hypnosis combined with relaxation (N = 4). Across interventions there was partial to moderate support for positive impact on measures of psychological well-being. Specific to relaxation, there was a lack of evidence to support any salutary effects of relaxation therapy alone on postsurgical outcomes; however, significant methodological problems cloud interpretation. For instance, in 6 studies (75%), patients were either given a relaxation audiotape or had a brief educational session on relaxation (10 minutes in one study, 40–70 minutes in another study) the day before surgery, which calls into question the possibility that the intervention was ill-timed, and did not allow sufficient time to practice and gain the relaxation skills required to affect the postsurgical recovery. In addition, studies tended to be nondirective (eg, "Listen to the CD as much as you want after surgery…"), and used a variety of measures and outcomes; the lack of standardization yielded some positive results but overall insufficient evidence that either a relaxation audio file/CD or brief relaxation delivered the day before surgery is beneficial.

The authors of the review reported that moderate evidence for guided imagery combined with relaxation and hypnosis combined with relaxation in improving surgical recovery. However, variability in methods used across studies limits interpretability and generalizability of findings. For instance, some studies included therapist contact, whereas others did not; some provided clear direction for practice and others did not. Across interventions, factors that seemed to be associated with greater efficacy included therapist contact and/or an educational session and specific directions regarding frequency of practice. To date, no reports have been found describing any presurgical interventions in hand surgery populations.

A notable omission from prior work is a combined relaxation and pain psychology approach, one that specifically targets pain-related anxiety and catastrophizing, provides pain education, and uses cognitive and behavioral strategies. Catastrophizing and pain-related anxiety are among the most mutable of all surgical risk factors (immutable factors include sex, age, trauma, and injury location). For this reason, pain psychology prehabilitation is an attractive option to potentially reduce postsurgical pain and improve function. Patients can increase their confidence in their ability to modulate their experience of pain by learning skills that improve the self-regulation of cognition, emotion, and physiologic hyperarousal. Functional MRI research has shown that use of such self-regulatory skills engages supraspinal structures and enhances descending noxious inhibitory pathways. Researchers of a functional MRI study conducted on healthy volunteers reported that a brief mindfulness intervention (totaling 80 minutes) effectively reduced pain intensity and pain unpleasantness in the evoked pain paradigm,[31] and that decreased pain was associated with reduced activation in regions of the brain associated with pain processing. Neuroimaging studies underscore the importance of cognition and attention in shaping individual differences in pain sensitivity.[32]

Recently, a single-session, 2-hour pain psychology class developed to specifically treating pain catastrophizing showed promise in outpatients with chronic pain. The brief intervention included specific psychoeducation regarding pain, catastrophizing, and self-regulation skills. Patients with chronic pain who underwent the brief pain catastrophizing group treatment (N = 57) had large treatment effects for reduced pain catastrophizing at 4 weeks posttreatment (Cohen $d = 1.15$).[33] Current studies are examining the feasibility and preliminary efficacy of this brief catastrophizing treatment tailored to the perioperative setting.

What does this mean to the hand surgeon? Despite empirical associations, practical questions remain regarding the clinical application of presurgical psychological screening using the Pain Catastrophizing Scale and the Pain Anxiety Symptom Scale.[34] In all studies discussed here, pain catastrophizing and pain-related anxiety were examined as continuous variables, with no studies providing guidance for cut-scores. Clearly, more research is needed to appropriately guide the referral of patients to perioperative pain psychology resources, particularly those who may show few outward signs of pain-related anxiety or psychological distress to the surgeon or other care providers but may still be experiencing both and thus unwittingly causing a negative impact on their surgical outcomes.

SUMMARY AND FUTURE DIRECTIONS

Associations across studies are not uniform, but there seems to be moderate evidence suggesting that presurgical pain catastrophizing and pain-related anxiety predict short-term and long-term outcomes for musculoskeletal surgery. Recent studies suggest that presurgical pain catastrophizing and pain-related anxiety predict recovery from hand surgery or trauma as indexed by pain and function. Results suggest that screening and treating pain-related distress may have salutary effects in surgical populations, including reductions in pain and opioid use, and increased function.

Recommendations for future research include the need to report and adjust for analgesic use in the study design. The practical utility of study findings may be improved by researchers reporting means for variables (vs correlations only), and by studies that risk-stratify patients and/or provide benchmarks to identify at-risk patients, thus informing referral to treatment. In addition, more research is needed regarding the efficacy of brief pain psychology treatment in the perioperative setting. Interpretability of findings may be improved with greater standardization in design of perioperative pain psychology treatment studies, including the selection of measures and in the timing of the intervention relative to the surgical procedure. Although the overall field is trending toward enhanced prehabilitation, pain psychology should be considered an integral component of multimodal care models. Pain psychology prehabilitation is a promising area of clinical research and care that stands to prepare patients to self-optimize their surgical outcomes.

REFERENCES

1. Sullivan MJ, Thorn B, Haythornthwaite JA, et al. Theoretical perspectives on the relation between catastrophizing and pain. Clin J Pain 2001;17(1): 52–64.
2. Keefe FJ, Brown GK, Wallston KA, et al. Coping with rheumatoid arthritis pain: catastrophizing as a maladaptive strategy. Pain 1989;37(1):51–6.
3. Sullivan MJL. The pain catastrophizing scale: development and validation. Psychol Assess 1995;7(4): 524–32.
4. Severeijns R, Vlaeyen JW, van den Hout MA, et al. Pain catastrophizing predicts pain intensity, disability, and psychological distress independent of the level of physical impairment. Clin J Pain 2001;17(2):165–72.
5. Papaioannou M, Skapinakis P, Damigos D, et al. The role of catastrophizing in the prediction of postoperative pain. Pain Med 2009;10(8):1452–9.
6. Pinto PR, McIntyre T, Almeida A, et al. The mediating role of pain catastrophizing in the relationship between presurgical anxiety and acute postsurgical pain after hysterectomy. Pain 2012;153(1):218–26.
7. Granot M, Ferber SG. The roles of pain catastrophizing and anxiety in the prediction of postoperative pain intensity: a prospective study. Clin J Pain 2005;21(5):439–45.
8. Weissman-Fogel I, Sprecher E, Pud D. Effects of catastrophizing on pain perception and pain modulation. Exp Brain Res 2008;186(1):79–85.
9. Martel MO, Wasan AD, Jamison RN, et al. Catastrophic thinking and increased risk for prescription opioid misuse in patients with chronic pain. Drug Alcohol Depend 2013;132(1–2):335–41.
10. Helmerhorst GT, Vranceanu AM, Vrahas M, et al. Risk factors for continued opioid use one to two months after surgery for musculoskeletal trauma. J Bone Joint Surg Am 2014;96(6):495–9.
11. Pinto PR, McIntyre T, Nogueira-Silva C, et al. Risk factors for persistent postsurgical pain in women undergoing hysterectomy due to benign causes: a prospective predictive study. J Pain 2012;13(11): 1045–57.
12. Wertli MM, Burgstaller JM, Weiser S, et al. The influence of catastrophizing on treatment outcome in patients with non-specific low back pain: a systematic review. Spine (Phila Pa 1976) 2013;39(3): 263–73.
13. Spinhoven P, Ter Kuile M, Kole-Snijders AM, et al. Catastrophizing and internal pain control as mediators of outcome in the multidisciplinary treatment of chronic low back pain. Eur J Pain 2004;8(3):211–9.
14. Abbott AD, Tyni-Lenne R, Hedlund R. Leg pain and psychological variables predict outcome 2-3 years after lumbar fusion surgery. Eur Spine J 2011; 20(10):1626–34.
15. Theunissen M, Peters ML, Bruce J, et al. Preoperative anxiety and catastrophizing: a systematic review and meta-analysis of the association with chronic postsurgical pain. Clin J Pain 2012;28(9):819–41.
16. George SZ, Wallace MR, Wright TW, et al. Evidence for a biopsychosocial influence on shoulder pain: pain catastrophizing and catechol-O-methyltransferase (COMT) diplotype predict clinical pain ratings. Pain 2008;136(1–2):53–61.
17. Vissers MM, Bussmann JB, Verhaar JA, et al. Psychological factors affecting the outcome of total hip and knee arthroplasty: a systematic review. Semin Arthritis Rheum 2012;41(4):576–88.
18. Bellamy N, Buchanan WW, Goldsmith CH, et al. Validation study of WOMAC: a health status instrument for measuring clinically important patient relevant outcomes to antirheumatic drug therapy in patients with osteoarthritis of the hip or knee. J Rheumatol 1988;15(12):1833–40.
19. Riddle DL, Wade JB, Jiranek WA, et al. Preoperative pain catastrophizing predicts pain outcome after knee arthroplasty. Clin Orthop Relat Res 2010; 468(3):798–806.
20. Vranceanu AM, Bachoura A, Weening A, et al. Psychological factors predict disability and pain intensity after skeletal trauma. J Bone Joint Surg Am 2014;96(3):e20.
21. McCracken LM, Dhingra L. A short version of the Pain Anxiety Symptoms Scale (PASS-20): preliminary development and validity. Pain Res Manag 2002;7(1):45–50.
22. Teunis T, Bot AG, Thornton ER, et al. Catastrophic thinking is associated with finger stiffness after distal radius fracture surgery. J Orthop Trauma 2015. [Epub ahead of print].
23. Roh YH, Lee BK, Noh JH, et al. Effect of anxiety and catastrophic pain ideation on early recovery after surgery for distal radius fractures. J Hand Surg Am 2014;39(11):2258–64.e2.
24. Keogh E, Book K, Thomas J, et al. Predicting pain and disability in patients with hand fractures: comparing pain anxiety, anxiety sensitivity and pain catastrophizing. Eur J Pain 2010;14(4): 446–51.
25. Connelly M, Fulmer RD, Prohaska J, et al. Predictors of postoperative pain trajectories in adolescent

idiopathic scoliosis. Spine (Phila Pa 1976) 2014; 39(3):E174–81.

26. Vranceanu AM, Jupiter JB, Mudgal CS, et al. Predictors of pain intensity and disability after minor hand surgery. J Hand Surg Am 2010;35(6):956–60.

27. Hudak PL, Amadio PC, Bombardier C. Development of an upper extremity outcome measure: the DASH (disabilities of the arm, shoulder and hand) [corrected]. The Upper Extremity Collaborative Group (UECG). Am J Ind Med 1996;29(6): 602–8.

28. Darnall BD. Less pain, fewer pills: avoid the dangers of prescription opioids and gain control over chronic pain. Boulder (CO): Bull Publishing; 2014.

29. Darnall BD. Enhanced pain management - binaural relaxation audio CD. Boulder (CO): Bull Publishing; 2014. Available at: https://www.bullpub.com/.

30. Nelson EA, Dowsey MM, Knowles SR, et al. Systematic review of the efficacy of pre-surgical mind-body based therapies on post-operative outcome measures. Complement Ther Med 2013;21(6):697–711.

31. Zeidan F, Martucci KT, Kraft RA, et al. Brain mechanisms supporting the modulation of pain by mindfulness meditation. J Neurosci 2011; 31(14):5540–8.

32. Emerson NM, Zeidan F, Lobanov OV, et al. Pain sensitivity is inversely related to regional grey matter density in the brain. Pain 2014;155(3):566–73.

33. Darnall BD, Sturgeon JA, Kao MC, et al. From catastrophizing to recovery: a pilot study of a single-session treatment for pain catastrophizing. J Pain Res 2014;14(7):219–26.

34. McCracken LM, Zayfert C, Gross RT. The Pain Anxiety Symptoms Scale: development and validation of a scale to measure fear of pain. Pain 1992; 50(1):67–73.

New Concepts in Complex Regional Pain Syndrome

Maral Tajerian, MSc, PhD[a,b], John David Clark, MD, PhD[a,b],*

KEYWORDS

- Complex regional pain syndrome • Preclinical models • Basic mechanisms • Neuroinflammation
- Autoimmunity • CNS plasticity • Disease progression

KEY POINTS

- Complex regional pain syndrome (CRPS) is initiated by dysfunction of the sympathetic nervous system as well as the release of neuropeptides released from afferent/effect c-fibers.
- Inflammatory mediators such as cytokines in peripheral tissues such as skin and muscle support CRPS-related pain.
- Autoimmunity may contribute to the manifestations of CRPS, although the immune targets are poorly understood.
- Biochemical and structural changes within the spinal cord and brain may explain the most persistent signs and symptoms of CRPS and may underlie the cognitive and emotional changes that accompany the syndrome.

INTRODUCTION

Complex regional pain syndrome (CRPS) is a painful, disabling, and often chronic condition that usually affects a single limb. With an estimated 50,000 new cases annually in the United States alone,[1] CRPS exhibits a higher prevalence in female patients, with women affected at least 3 times more than men.[1] The most frequent causes of CRPS involve surgery and trauma, with hand surgery being a particularly relevant factor; for example, the rate of CRPS is 5% to 40% after fasciectomy for Dupuytren contracture,[2] 8% after carpal tunnel surgery,[3] and greater than 30% after distal radius fracture.[4] Interestingly, the likelihood of developing CRPS is not proportional to the extent of injury or surgery, because it can occur after even very minor injuries[5] In addition, limb immobilization itself appears to be a risk factor for development of this condition.[6,7]

Although acute CRPS sometimes improves with early and aggressive physical therapy, CRPS present for a period of 1 year or greater rarely spontaneously resolves,[8] thus leaving the majority (80%) of patients severely disabled.[9] The syndrome encompasses a disparate collection of signs and symptoms involving the sensory, motor, and autonomic nervous systems, cognitive deficits, changes in mood, anxiety, bone demineralization, skin growth changes, and vascular dysfunction. Despite the devastating nature of the syndrome, to date, no satisfactory treatments exist for the CRPS patient, mainly due to the heterogeneity of the patient population, the evolving nature of the syndrome, and the overall lack of understanding of its basic underlying mechanisms.

Funding Sources: N/A (Dr M. Tajerian); supported by National Institutes of Health grant R01NS072143 and Veterans Affairs Merit Review grant I01RX001475 (Dr J.D. Clark).
Conflict of Interest: Nil.
a Anesthesia Service, Veterans Affairs Palo Alto Health Care System, 3801 Miranda Avenue, Palo Alto, CA 94304, USA; b Department of Anesthesiology, Stanford University School of Medicine, 300 Pasteur Drive, Stanford, CA 94305, USA
* Corresponding author. Anesthesia Service, Veterans Affairs Palo Alto Health Care System, 3801 Miranda Avenue, Palo Alto, CA 94304.
E-mail address: djclark@stanford.edu

Multifaceted disorders, including CRPS, are often difficult to explain by a single core mechanism. The current review addresses recent developments in understanding the various mechanisms underlying CRPS using data from preclinical models as well as clinical studies (for a summary, please see **Fig. 1**). Pursuing these mechanisms will be key to understanding the vulnerability of some surgical and trauma patients to CRPS as well as inspiring mechanism-based treatments that go beyond simple symptom management.

ANIMAL MODELS OF COMPLEX REGIONAL PAIN SYNDROME

Animal models reflecting different aspects of CRPS have been invaluable to exploring some of the basic mechanisms of the syndrome. These models include the following:

a. Peripheral nerve injury: One of the earliest described models of CRPS, it relies on induced nerve injury to reproduce some of the clinical symptoms of spontaneous pain, hyperalgesia, and limb edema.[10]
b. Ischemia/reperfusion injury: Developed in rats over a decade ago,[11] this model is based on clinical observations showing ischemic signs in CRPS patients, including decreased levels of hemoglobin oxygenation in skin capillaries,[12] increased anaerobic glycolysis,[13,14] and decreased skin blood flow.[15] This model also has been shown to exhibit altered expression of cerebral proteins.[16]

c. Limb trauma and immobilization: Characterized in both mice[17] and rats,[18] this model focuses on the surgery/trauma causes of CRPS and mimics many of the nociceptive and vascular changes observed in humans in the acute and chronic stages of the syndrome.
d. Limb immobilization: Similar to clinical experiments wherein limb immobilization is associated with transient nociceptive hypersensitivity,[7] this general model of chronic widespread pain focuses on limb immobilization and potentially tight cast application, as the causative agent of CRPS in rats.[19]

It is notable that most currently used models rely on physical trauma to the rodent hindpaw, in an effort to mimic injuries shown in CRPS patients, including fractures, strains, tight application of casts, and other traumas. Common to other animal models, none of these models accurately mimics all symptoms experienced by CRPS patients, a notoriously heterogeneous population. Nonetheless, these models reproduce many of the key characteristics of CRPS and allow the study of the molecular details of the disorder as well as the testing of new treatment strategies. The next few paragraphs address some of the recent advances in the understanding of the mechanisms of CRPS in both preclinical models and clinical subjects.

SYMPATHETIC NERVOUS SYSTEM

Although the term "reflex sympathetic dystrophy" has been replaced by the less mechanistically presumptive CRPS, there is evidence supporting the

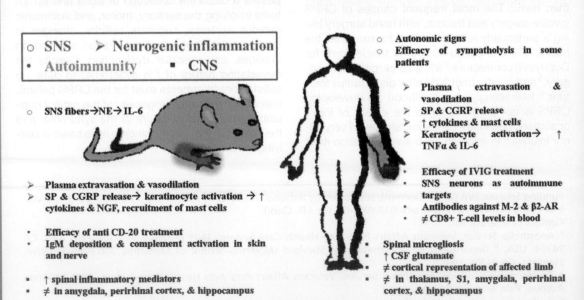

Fig. 1. Summary of some of the basic mechanisms involved in CRPS in preclinical models and patients. CSF, cerebrospinal fluid; M-2, muscarinic acetylcholine receptor 2; NE, norepinephrine; S1, primary somatosensory cortex.

role of the sympathetic nervous system (SNS) in the development and maintenance of the syndrome. Historically, this role was inferred based on autonomic physical signs and on symptom relief following sympatholysis.[20] More recent studies have proposed that sympathetic dysfunction coincides with the onset of the disease but normalizes with time,[21] suggesting a role in the genesis of CRPS rather than its maintenance, although additional studies have revealed significant SNS dysfunction in many chronic CRPS patients.[22] In the rat tibia fracture model of CRPS, it was demonstrated that sympathetic fibers release norepinephrine, which in turn stimulates interleukin (IL)-6 production, supporting the observed CRPS-like changes. More detailed in vitro studies revealed β-2 adrenergic receptors (β2-AR) to be the receptor population mainly responsible for the liberation of IL-6.[23] The upregulation of α-1 adrenergic receptors in skin samples from CRPS patients suggests there is also a role for this receptor population as well.[24] Thus, there are several clinical and molecular clues pointing to the role of SNS in CRPS.

Despite evidence showing the involvement of SNS in the pathophysiology of CRPS, the direct link between SNS activity and nociception remains to be delineated in CRPS patients: for example, in a study examining 24 CRPS patients and using microneurography techniques, no links were found between efferent fiber sympathetic activity and afferent activity in nociceptors innervating the symptomatic areas.[25] These findings might suggest that indirect mechanisms could be responsible for both the activation and the sensitization of nociceptors, not a direct coupling. One such mechanism could be due to a notable symptom of CRPS, vasoconstriction, which could influence nociceptor microenvironment or activate macrophages, which in turn would result in inflammatory mediator release.[26]

Based on the principle that there is some aspect of sympathetically maintained pain in CRPS, it stands to reason that sympatholysis should be efficacious in reversing some of the peripheral sensitization observed in CRPS patients. However, evidence remains mixed for both regional (local block of noradrenaline from sympathetic fibers) and proximal (at the sympathetic ganglion) treatment studies.[27] This lack of efficacy does not necessarily indicate the absence of SNS involvement, but could be due to the heterogeneity of the patient population, whereby only a subset of CRPS sufferers displays sympathetically maintained pain.

NEUROGENIC INFLAMMATION

There are 2 major components of neurogenic inflammation: plasma extravasation and vasodilation.[28]

CRPS is characterized by changes in blood flow, limb temperature, and edema in both humans[13,29] and rodent models.[11,18] Biochemically, neurogenic inflammation is characterized by the release of Substance P (SP) and calcitonin gene-related peptide (CGRP) from afferent neurons.[28] Evidence from both CRPS patients and laboratory animals suggests that, in the early stage of CRPS often known clinically as the warm phase, primary afferent C-fibers and sympathetic neurons function aberrantly, resulting in vascular symptoms, trophic changes, and pain.[30] In the rodent tibial fracture/cast model of CRPS, it has been shown that neuropeptides such as SP and CGRP released from sensory c-fibers lead to pain sensitization by the activation of receptors on keratinocytes and vascular endothelial cells, causing the local production of high levels of cytokines and nerve growth factor (NGF)[31–34] as well as the recruitment of mediator-rich mast cells.[35]

Similar observations showed increased levels of secreted cytokines, including tumor necrosis factor-α (TNF-α) and IL-6, in studies conducted in blister suction samples acquired from CRPS patients.[36–38] Likewise, TNF-α and other pronociceptive cytokines were identified at elevated levels in the skin of CRPS patients[36,38–40] and postsurgical patients with persistent limb pain,[41] as were mast cells, cells capable of releasing a host of nociceptive and vasoactive mediators.[42] Recent studies using skin biopsies from acute and chronic CRPS patients demonstrated that cytokine levels drop and mast cell infiltration resolves as the condition becomes more chronic.[43] Finally, similar to what was seen in the rodent model, keratinocyte activation and proliferation were reported in CRPS skin and shown to be associated with upregulated levels of TNF-α and IL-6.[43]

These observations of alterations at the molecular level could provide a basis for mechanism-based treatments. For instance, antineuropeptide signaling and anti-mast cell agents might both prove to be of therapeutic value for CRPS, by antagonizing neuropeptide receptors[44] and affecting the division and degranulation of mast cells.[45] Similarly, peripherally restricted biologic anti-TNF-α agents, such as infliximab, may be effective in reducing pain in CRPS, although this therapy might be most efficacious in acute CRPS when peripheral TNF-α levels are highest.[46] Despite the availability of such agents, the published evidence remains preliminary. For instance, although a case study in a CRPS patient showed pain amelioration and improvement in the cutaneous dystrophic symptoms after systemic infliximab administration,[47] a double-blind, randomized, placebo-controlled study of the efficacy infliximab in CRPS was discontinued due to budgetary limitations even though a trend toward drug efficacy was observed.[48] Clinical trials involving anti-IL-1β and IL-6 are unavailable at this point. Finally, although not a selective immunosuppressant, prednisone used in a short course does seem to have efficacy in speeding the resolution of CRPS.[49] Modulation of the neurogenic inflammation pathways remains an important area of focus to improve care of the CRPS patient.

AUTOIMMUNITY

A collection of observations made over the past decade suggests an autoimmune cause for CRPS, a hypothesis that would help explain the seemingly unrelated nature of the syndrome's signs and symptoms as well as difficulties in achieving adequate symptom control, remission, or cure using standard therapies. Exploration of CRPS-related autoimmunity began with the opportune observation of symptom improvement in CRPS patients treated with intravenous immunoglobulin (IVIG) for unrelated conditions. This observation was followed by an exploratory clinical trial[50] and later a randomized trial of low-dose IVIG showing intermediate duration (3 months) control of long-standing CRPS symptoms in many patients.[51] These findings were further explored in an animal model, where immunoglobulin G (IgG) from CRPS patients was shown to worsen nociceptive sensitization in laboratory animals undergoing mild tissue trauma.[52] Similarly, CRPS-like symptoms following fracture/cast immobilization were shown to be less severe in mice treated with anti-CD20 (rituximab) and in mu-MT mice (lacking mature B cells) compared with wild-type (WT) mice that had undergone the same procedure. Furthermore, immunoglobulin M (IgM) deposition and complement activation were observed in the skin and sciatic nerves of WT fracture/cast mice.[53]

Clinically, the autoimmune hypothesis was bolstered by 2 additional sets of observations. First, it was demonstrated that a disproportionate number of patients had IgM and IgG profiles consistent with antecedent infections by chlamydia, parvovirus, and campylobacter.[54,55] Cross-reactivity of infection-related antibodies with self-antigens is thought to explain some cases of autoimmune neuropathy. Second, experiments using immunohistochemical techniques and fluorescence-assisted cell sorting analysis identified SNS neurons as targets for autoantibodies from some CRPS patients with little evidence of such autoimmunity from patients with other types of peripheral neuropathy.[55,56] Follow-up experiments using in vitro beating cardiomyocyte preparations suggested that most CRPS, but not healthy, patients had autoantibodies binding to and activating the M-2 muscarinic and the β2-AR.[57] Interestingly, there are other patients without pain who produce anti-β-2-AR antibodies, but their symptoms are orthostatic hypotension, suggesting that autoantibody expression alone may not be sufficient to cause CRPS.[35,58] Importantly, the authors have recently provided evidence suggesting that β2-ARs are critical to CRPS-like changes in the fracture/cast model.[23] Additional evidence for autoimmune mechanisms in CRPS includes genetic data supporting CRPS associations with specific human leukocyte antigens,[59–61] studies showing altered CD8+ T-cell levels in peripheral blood, and case reports of Langerhans antigen-presenting cell proliferation in the skin of CRPS patients.[62]

Approaching CRPS as an autoimmune disease opens entirely new experimental pathways to identifying specific supporting mechanisms and provides opportunities for novel therapeutic development. Further exploration of CRPS-related autoimmunity may help to provide a rational basis for the use of treatments such as IVIG, anti-CD20 (rituximab), or other clinically available immunotherapies. These treatments are disease-modifying rather than being directed toward providing analgesia. Some, like the use of steroids, are suitable for perioperative use, whereas others, such as strong and persistent immune modulators, may be best reserved as second- and third-line agents. Indeed, the adverse consequences of persistent immunosuppression may limit the utility of some of these therapies.

CENTRAL NERVOUS SYSTEM CHANGES

Several manifestations of CRPS suggest functional changes within the central nervous system (CNS), including motor changes, autonomic functions, and changes in cortical representation. Motor symptoms have been identified in up to 97% of CRPS patients and include phenomena such as exaggerated tendon reflexes, dystonia, myoclonus, paresis, and tremor; changes thought to rely in large part on CNS dysfunction.[13] Further evidence of CNS involvement comes from a case report of spinal microgliosis in a cadaveric CRPS subject[63] and increased levels of glutamate in the cerebrospinal fluid of CRPS patients.[64] In the fracture model of CRPS, nociceptive sensitization is supported by increased expression of spinal inflammatory mediators (TNF-α, IL-1β, IL-6, chemokine (C-C motif) ligand 2 [CCL2], NGF) that are upregulated by spinal neuropeptides (SP, CGRP) signaling.[65] The intrathecal administration of selective receptor antagonists for SP, CGRP, TNF-α, IL-1β, IL-6, CCL2, or NGF ameliorated pain sensitivity in these animals.[65]

In addition to alterations at the level of the spinal cord, functional, anatomic, and biochemical changes are observed in the brain and are associated with altered behavior in both rodents and humans. In the fracture model of CRPS, signs of anxiety and memory impairment are accompanied by structural and biochemical changes in the amygdala, perirhinal cortex, and hippocampus,[66] including changes in dendritic complexity and levels of brain-derived neurotrophic factor and synaptophysin in these regions. In CRPS patients, cortical representation of involved limbs is altered[67,68] and is correlated with central pain sensitization.[69] Furthermore, clear alterations in cognition, memory, and emotions (anxiety and depression) in CRPS sufferers have been demonstrated,[70–75] potentially due to diminished GABAergic or N-methyl-D–aspartate–mediated cortical neuroplasticity.[76] It is notable that these changes seem to be reversible: for instance, ketamine treatment was associated with improved CRPS symptoms as well as improvements in cognition.[77]

Finally, neuroimaging studies have identified CRPS-associated changes in several centers including thalamus, S1, and S2 (somatosensory processing), cingulate and amygdala (emotion functioning), hippocampus and perirhinal regions (memory functioning), and other regions as well as the connectivity between these centers.[69,78–86] Imaging studies in children demonstrate that some CRPS-related brain structural and functional changes resolve in parallel with symptom resolution, supporting a functional link between these areas and functions, while other areas remain altered, providing a basis for the increased susceptibility to recurrent CRPS known to exist in these patients.[87,88]

Together, these data emphasize the importance of studying the central correlates of CRPS that could be responsible for the chronification of the symptoms, in addition to inspiring therapeutic interventions that do not necessarily target peripheral mechanisms, but attempt to ameliorate the broader pain experience by targeting its associated cognitive and emotional comorbidities.

ACUTE VERSUS CHRONIC COMPLEX REGIONAL PAIN SYNDROME

Given the changing nature of CRPS over time, it is of great importance to understand the aforementioned mechanisms within the acute and chronic time frames of the syndrome. In CRPS patients, the clinical signs and symptoms seem to be of a dynamic nature, where the impacted limb evolves from an acute warm phase (limb is sensitive, is swollen, and displays an elevated temperature) to a chronic cold phase (resolution of inflamed appearance, but the persistence of pain and disability).[13] More generally, the evolution of the syndrome is characterized by the transition from an acute state with prominent peripheral features to a chronic form characterized by persistent pain along with significant cognitive and mood changes.[30,89–91]

To date, the fracture/cast rodent model of CRPS is the only animal model wherein the acute versus chronic time points were explored using behavioral and molecular tools. This model showed that although mechanical allodynia persists for a long time, it is only at the acute stage that mice exhibit signs of edema and increased hindpaw temperature. These early symptoms are accompanied by the upregulation of various molecules involved in chemokine signaling pathways.[92] Furthermore, similar to the clinical population, pain-related cognitive, emotional, and neuroplastic alterations are observed in the chronic stages in the preclinical model.[66]

In addition to providing a more comprehensive view of disease cause, studying the evolution of CRPS is crucial in determining the choice of treatment. For instance, pinpointing the mechanisms behind the early stages (such as the inflammatory and immunologic aspects) might suggest novel approaches to preventing the occurrence of CRPS as well as halting and reversing the condition at its earliest stages. Conversely, mechanisms unique to the chronic stage (such as central sensitization) might suggest therapies directed toward already-established CRPS. In a recent study conducted in the fracture model of CRPS, chronic ketamine infusions were efficacious when administered in the chronic, but not acute phase of the syndrome,[93] suggesting that this centrally directed therapy be used in patients with longer-established CRPS.

SUMMARY

CRPS, once entirely enigmatic, is now appreciated to have a complex and evolving basis. Although mechanisms such as SNS dysfunction and neurogenic inflammation have long been known to regulate the vascular, trophic, and pain-related features of the syndrome, the novel concept of autoimmune involvement is becoming increasingly associated with complex syndromes including CRPS. The recent realization that changes within the CNS may underlie the most chronic sensory features of CRPS as well as the associated psychological changes also opens the door to the development of new treatments. Taken together, these recent advances in CRPS support the optimistic view that new treatments might be rationally designed based on disease cause and applied to individual patients based on their particular CRPS-related signs and symptoms.[26]

REFERENCES

1. de Mos M, de Bruijn AG, Huygen FJ, et al. The incidence of complex regional pain syndrome: a population-based study. Pain 2007;129:12–20.

2. Reuben SS. Chronic pain after surgery: what can we do to prevent it. Curr Pain Headache Rep 2007;11: 5–13.

3. da Costa VV, de Oliveira SB, Fernandes Mdo C, et al. Incidence of regional pain syndrome after carpal tunnel release. Is there a correlation with the anesthetic technique? Rev Bras Anestesiol 2011; 61:425–33.

4. Atkins RM, Tindale W, Bickerstaff D, et al. Quantitative bone scintigraphy in reflex sympathetic dystrophy. Br J Rheumatol 1993;32:41–5.

5. Veldman PH, Reynen HM, Arntz IE, et al. Signs and symptoms of reflex sympathetic dystrophy: prospective study of 829 patients. Lancet 1993;342:1012–6.

6. Allen G, Galer BS, Schwartz L. Epidemiology of complex regional pain syndrome: a retrospective chart review of 134 patients. Pain 1999;80:539–44.

7. Terkelsen AJ, Bach FW, Jensen TS. Experimental forearm immobilization in humans induces cold and mechanical hyperalgesia. Anesthesiology 2008;109: 297–307.

8. Schwartzman RJ, Erwin KL, Alexander GM. The natural history of complex regional pain syndrome. Clin J Pain 2009;25:273–80.

9. Subbarao J, Stillwell GK. Reflex sympathetic dystrophy syndrome of the upper extremity: analysis of total outcome of management of 125 cases. Arch Phys Med Rehabil 1981;62:549–54.

10. Kingery WS, Guo T, Agashe GS, et al. Glucocorticoid inhibition of neuropathic limb edema and cutaneous neurogenic extravasation. Brain Res 2001;913:140–8.

11. Coderre TJ, Xanthos DN, Francis L, et al. Chronic post-ischemia pain (CPIP): a novel animal model of complex regional pain syndrome-type I (CRPS-I; reflex sympathetic dystrophy) produced by prolonged hindpaw ischemia and reperfusion in the rat. Pain 2004;112:94–105.

12. Koban M, Leis S, Schultze-Mosgau S, et al. Tissue hypoxia in complex regional pain syndrome. Pain 2003;104:149–57.

13. Birklein F, Riedl B, Sieweke N, et al. Neurological findings in complex regional pain syndromes– analysis of 145 cases. Acta Neurol Scand 2000; 101:262–9.

14. Birklein F, Weber M, Neundorfer B. Increased skin lactate in complex regional pain syndrome: evidence for tissue hypoxia? Neurology 2000;55:1213–5.

15. Kurvers HA, Jacobs MJ, Beuk RJ, et al. Reflex sympathetic dystrophy: evolution of microcirculatory disturbances in time. Pain 1995;60:333–40.

16. Nahm FS, Park ZY, Nahm SS, et al. Proteomic identification of altered cerebral proteins in the complex regional pain syndrome animal model. Biomed Res Int 2014;2014:498410.

17. Guo TZ, Wei T, Shi X, et al. Neuropeptide deficient mice have attenuated nociceptive, vascular, and inflammatory changes in a tibia fracture model of complex regional pain syndrome. Mol Pain 2012;8:85.

18. Guo TZ, Offley SC, Boyd EA, et al. Substance P signaling contributes to the vascular and nociceptive abnormalities observed in a tibial fracture rat model of complex regional pain syndrome type I. Pain 2004;108:95–107.

19. Ohmichi M, Ohmichi Y, Ohishi H, et al. Activated spinal astrocytes are involved in the maintenance of chronic widespread mechanical hyperalgesia after cast immobilization. Mol Pain 2014;10:6.

20. Loh L, Nathan PW. Painful peripheral states and sympathetic blocks. J Neurol Neurosurg Psychiatr 1978;41:664–71.

21. Gradl G, Schurmann M. Sympathetic dysfunction as a temporary phenomenon in acute posttraumatic CRPS I. Clin Auton Res 2005;15:29–34.

22. Vogel T, Gradl G, Ockert B, et al. Sympathetic dysfunction in long-term complex regional pain syndrome. Clin J Pain 2010;26:128–31.

23. Li W, Shi X, Wang L, et al. Epidermal adrenergic signaling contributes to inflammation and pain sensitization in a rat model of complex regional pain syndrome. Pain 2013;154:1224–36.

24. Drummond PD, Drummond ES, Dawson LF, et al. Upregulation of α1-adrenoceptors on cutaneous nerve fibres after partial sciatic nerve ligation and in complex regional pain syndrome type II. Pain 2014;155:606–16.

25. Campero M, Bostock H, Baumann TK, et al. A search for activation of C nociceptors by sympathetic fibers in complex regional pain syndrome. Clin Neurophysiol 2010;121:1072–9.

26. Gierthmuhlen J, Binder A, Baron R. Mechanism-based treatment in complex regional pain syndromes. Nat Rev Neurol 2014;10:518–28.

27. Kingery WS. A critical review of controlled clinical trials for peripheral neuropathic pain and complex regional pain syndromes. Pain 1997;73:123–39.

28. Birklein F, Schmelz M. Neuropeptides, neurogenic inflammation and complex regional pain syndrome (CRPS). Neurosci Lett 2008;437:199–202.

29. Birklein F, Riedl B, Claus D, et al. Pattern of autonomic dysfunction in time course of complex

regional pain syndrome. Clin Auton Res 1998;8: 79–85.

30. Bruehl S. An update on the pathophysiology of complex regional pain syndrome. Anesthesiology 2010; 113:713–25.

31. Li WW, Guo TZ, Li XQ, et al. Fracture induces keratinocyte activation, proliferation, and expression of pro-nociceptive inflammatory mediators. Pain 2010; 151:843–52.

32. Li WW, Sabsovich I, Guo TZ, et al. The role of enhanced cutaneous IL-1beta signaling in a rat tibia fracture model of complex regional pain syndrome. Pain 2009;144:303–13.

33. Sabsovich I, Guo TZ, Wei T, et al. TNF signaling contributes to the development of nociceptive sensitization in a tibia fracture model of complex regional pain syndrome type I. Pain 2008;137:507–19.

34. Sabsovich I, Wei T, Guo TZ, et al. Effect of anti-NGF antibodies in a rat tibia fracture model of complex regional pain syndrome type I. Pain 2008;138: 47–60.

35. Li WW, Guo TZ, Liang DY, et al. Substance P signaling controls mast cell activation, degranulation, and nociceptive sensitization in a rat fracture model of complex regional pain syndrome. Anesthesiology 2012;116:882–95.

36. Groeneweg JG, Huygen FJ, Heijmans-Antonissen C, et al. Increased endothelin-1 and diminished nitric oxide levels in blister fluids of patients with intermediate cold type complex regional pain syndrome type 1. BMC Musculoskelet Disord 2006;7:91.

37. Heijmans-Antonissen C, Wesseldijk F, Munnikes RJ, et al. Multiplex bead array assay for detection of 25 soluble cytokines in blister fluid of patients with complex regional pain syndrome type 1. Mediators Inflamm 2006;2006:28398.

38. Huygen FJ, De Bruijn AG, De Bruin MT, et al. Evidence for local inflammation in complex regional pain syndrome type 1. Mediators Inflamm 2002;11: 47–51.

39. Munnikes RJ, Muis C, Boersma M, et al. Intermediate stage complex regional pain syndrome type 1 is unrelated to proinflammatory cytokines. Mediators Inflamm 2005;2005:366–72.

40. Pepper A, Li W, Kingery WS, et al. Complex regional pain syndrome-like changes following surgery and immobilization. J Pain 2013;14(5):516–24.

41. Pepper A, Li W, Kingery WS, et al. Changes resembling complex regional pain syndrome following surgery and immobilization. J Pain 2013;14:516–24.

42. Huygen FJ, Ramdhani N, van Toorenenbergen A, et al. Mast cells are involved in inflammatory reactions during Complex Regional Pain Syndrome type 1. Immunol Lett 2004;91:147–54.

43. Birklein F, Drummond PD, Li W, et al. Activation of cutaneous immune responses in complex regional pain syndrome. J Pain 2014;15:485–95.

44. Wei T, Guo TZ, Li WW, et al. Keratinocyte expression of inflammatory mediators plays a crucial role in substance P-induced acute and chronic pain. J Neuroinflammation 2012;9:181.

45. Dirckx M, Groeneweg G, van Daele PL, et al. Mast cells: a new target in the treatment of complex regional pain syndrome? Pain Pract 2013;13: 599–603.

46. Bernateck M, Karst M, Gratz KF, et al. The first scintigraphic detection of tumor necrosis factor-alpha in patients with complex regional pain syndrome type 1. Anesth Analg 2010;110:211–5.

47. Miclescu AA, Nordquist L, Hysing EB, et al. Targeting oxidative injury and cytokines' activity in the treatment with anti-tumor necrosis factor-αantibody for complex regional pain syndrome 1. Pain Pract 2013;13:641–8.

48. Dirckx M, Groeneweg G, Wesseldijk F, et al. Report of a preliminary discontinued double-blind, randomized, placebo-controlled trial of the anti-TNF-αchimeric monoclonal antibody infliximab in complex regional pain syndrome. Pain Pract 2013;13:633–40.

49. Christensen K, Jensen EM, Noer I. The reflex dystrophy syndrome response to treatment with systemic corticosteroids. Acta Chir Scand 1982;148:653–5.

50. Goebel A, Blaes F. Complex regional pain syndrome, prototype of a novel kind of autoimmune disease. Autoimmun Rev 2013;12(6):682–6.

51. Goebel A, Baranowski A, Maurer K, et al. Intravenous immunoglobulin treatment of the complex regional pain syndrome: a randomized trial. Ann Intern Med 2010;152:152–8.

52. Tekus V, Hajna Z, Borbely E, et al. A CRPS-IgG-transfer-trauma model reproducing inflammatory and positive sensory signs associated with complex regional pain syndrome. Pain 2014;155:299–308.

53. Li WW, Guo TZ, Shi X, et al. Autoimmunity contributes to nociceptive sensitization in a mouse model of complex regional pain syndrome. Pain 2014; 155:2377–89.

54. Goebel A. Screening of patients with complex regional pain syndrome for antecedent infections. Clin J Pain 2001;17:378–9.

55. Goebel A, Vogel H, Caneris O, et al. Immune responses to Campylobacter and serum autoantibodies in patients with complex regional pain syndrome. J Neuroimmunol 2005;162:184–9.

56. Kohr D, Tschernatsch M, Schmitz K, et al. Autoantibodies in complex regional pain syndrome bind to a differentiation-dependent neuronal surface autoantigen. Pain 2009;143:246–51.

57. Kohr D, Singh P, Tschernatsch M, et al. Autoimmunity against the β2 adrenergic receptor and muscarinic-2 receptor in complex regional pain syndrome. Pain 2011;152:2690–700.

58. Yu X, Stavrakis S, Hill MA, et al. Autoantibody activation of beta-adrenergic and muscarinic receptors

contributes to an "autoimmune" orthostatic hypotension. J Am Soc Hypertens 2012;6:40–7.

59. de Rooij AM, Florencia Gosso M, Haasnoot GW, et al. HLA-B62 and HLA-DQ8 are associated with complex regional pain syndrome with fixed dystonia. Pain 2009;145:82–5.

60. van de Beek WJ, Roep BO, van der Slik AR, et al. Susceptibility loci for complex regional pain syndrome. Pain 2003;103:93–7.

61. van Rooijen DE, Roelen DL, Verduijn W, et al. Genetic HLA associations in complex regional pain syndrome with and without dystonia. J Pain 2012;13:784–9.

62. Calder JS, Holten I, McAllister RM. Evidence for immune system involvement in reflex sympathetic dystrophy. J Hand Surg 1998;23:147–50.

63. Del Valle L, Schwartzman RJ, Alexander G. Spinal cord histopathological alterations in a patient with longstanding complex regional pain syndrome. Brain Behav Immun 2009;23:85–91.

64. Alexander GM, Perreault MJ, Reichenberger ER, et al. Changes in immune and glial markers in the CSF of patients with complex regional pain syndrome. Brain Behav Immun 2007;21:668–76.

65. Shi X, Guo T, Wei T, et al. Facilitated spinal neuropeptide signaling and upregulated inflammatory mediator expression contributes to post-fracture nociceptive sensitization. Pain 2015.

66. Tajerian M, Leu D, Zou Y, et al. Brain neuroplastic changes accompany anxiety and memory deficits in a model of complex regional pain syndrome. Anesthesiology 2014;121:852–65.

67. Moseley GL, Wiech K. The effect of tactile discrimination training is enhanced when patients watch the reflected image of their unaffected limb during training. Pain 2009;144:314–9.

68. Pleger B, Tegenthoff M, Ragert P, et al. Sensorimotor retuning [corrected] in complex regional pain syndrome parallels pain reduction. Ann Neurol 2005; 57:425–9.

69. Vartiainen NV, Kirveskari E, Forss N. Central processing of tactile and nociceptive stimuli in complex regional pain syndrome. Clin Neurophysiol 2008; 119:2380–8.

70. Apkarian AV, Sosa Y, Krauss BR, et al. Chronic pain patients are impaired on an emotional decision-making task. Pain 2004;108:129–36.

71. Maihofner C, DeCol R. Decreased perceptual learning ability in complex regional pain syndrome. Eur J Pain 2007;11:903–9.

72. Libon DJ, Schwartzman RJ, Eppig J, et al. Neuropsychological deficits associated with complex regional pain syndrome. J Int Neuropsychol Soc 2010;16:566–73.

73. Dilek B, Yemez B, Kizil R, et al. Anxious personality is a risk factor for developing complex regional pain syndrome type I. Rheumatol Int 2012;32: 915–20.

74. Harden RN, Bruehl S, Perez RS, et al. Development of a severity score for CRPS. Pain 2010; 151:870–6.

75. Lohnberg JA, Altmaier EM. A review of psychosocial factors in complex regional pain syndrome. J Clin Psychol Med Settings 2013;20(2):247–54.

76. Dinse HR, Ragert P, Pleger B, et al. Pharmacological modulation of perceptual learning and associated cortical reorganization. Science 2003;301:91–4.

77. Koffler SP, Hampstead BM, Irani F, et al. The neurocognitive effects of 5 day anesthetic ketamine for the treatment of refractory complex regional pain syndrome. Arch Clin Neuropsychol 2007;22: 719–29.

78. Baliki MN, Schnitzer TJ, Bauer WR, et al. Brain morphological signatures for chronic pain. PLoS One 2011;6:e26010.

79. Becerra L, Schwartzman RJ, Kiefer RT, et al. CNS measures of pain responses pre- and post-anesthetic ketamine in a patient with complex regional pain syndrome. Pain Med 2009. [Epub ahead of print].

80. Freund W, Wunderlich AP, Stuber G, et al. The role of periaqueductal gray and cingulate cortex during suppression of pain in complex regional pain syndrome. Clin J Pain 2011;27:796–804.

81. Geha PY, Baliki MN, Harden RN, et al. The brain in chronic CRPS pain: abnormal gray-white matter interactions in emotional and autonomic regions. Neuron 2008;60:570–81.

82. Grachev ID, Thomas PS, Ramachandran TS. Decreased levels of N-acetylaspartate in dorsolateral prefrontal cortex in a case of intractable severe sympathetically mediated chronic pain (complex regional pain syndrome, type I). Brain Cogn 2002; 49:102–13.

83. Maihofner C, Forster C, Birklein F, et al. Brain processing during mechanical hyperalgesia in complex regional pain syndrome: a functional MRI study. Pain 2005;114:93–103.

84. Maihofner C, Handwerker HO, Birklein F. Functional imaging of allodynia in complex regional pain syndrome. Neurology 2006;66:711–7.

85. Maihofner C, Handwerker HO, Neundorfer B, et al. Patterns of cortical reorganization in complex regional pain syndrome. Neurology 2003;61:1707–15.

86. Maihofner C, Seifert F, Markovic K. Complex regional pain syndromes: new pathophysiological concepts and therapies. Eur J Neurol 2010;17:649–60.

87. Lebel A, Becerra L, Wallin D, et al. fMRI reveals distinct CNS processing during symptomatic and recovered complex regional pain syndrome in children. Brain 2008;131:1854–79.

88. Linnman C, Becerra L, Lebel A, et al. Transient and persistent pain induced connectivity alterations in pediatric complex regional pain syndrome. PLoS One 2013;8:e57205.

89. Bean DJ, Johnson MH, Kydd RR. The outcome of complex regional pain syndrome type 1: a systematic review. J Pain 2014;15:677–90.

90. Bean DJ, Johnson MH, Kydd RR. Relationships between psychological factors, pain, and disability in complex regional pain syndrome and low back pain. Clin J Pain 2014;30:647–53.

91. Eberle T, Doganci B, Kramer HH, et al. Warm and cold complex regional pain syndromes: differences beyond skin temperature? Neurology 2009;72:505–12.

92. Gallagher JJ, Tajerian M, Guo T, et al. Acute and chronic phases of complex regional pain syndrome in mice are accompanied by distinct transcriptional changes in the spinal cord. Mol Pain 2013;9:40.

90. Tajerian M, Leu D, Yang P, et al. Differential efficacy of ketamine in the acute versus chronic stages of complex regional pain syndrome in mice. Anesthesiology 2015.

Pharmacologic Management of Upper Extremity Chronic Nerve Pain

Ian Carroll, MD, MS

KEYWORDS

- Chronic pain • Neuropathic • Nerve • Tricyclic • Gabapentin • Postsurgical

KEY POINTS

- Chronic pain complicates all types of surgery, including upper extremity surgery done with excellent technique.
- Chronic postsurgical pain is usually neuropathic even though it is not described as burning or electrical but is more commonly described as deep and throbbing.
- Cutaneous neuromas (scar neuromas) are common and can only be excluded by injecting the scar.
- Medication management tailored to neuropathic pain is often effective and the principles of such management are outlined in the article.

Chronic pain following surgery is a major complication affecting between 10% and 30% of patients following a wide variety of surgeries.[1] The hand and upper limb are especially susceptible to postsurgical pain because of the rich innervation and unique demands of the upper extremity. Neuropathic pain after hand/upper limb surgery is likely produced through at least 3 potential mechanisms: (1) transection of cutaneous branches during skin incision with neuroma formation in the skin scar[2-5]; (2) adherence of postsurgical scar tissue to nerves either in the skin or deeper without transection of these nerves (exacerbated by the postoperative immobilization often required for bone healing)[6]; and (3) entrapment of nerve branches remote from the skin incision. This entrapment can be proximal to the surgical insult caused by edema tracking along the nerve course and resulting in compression at sites where surrounding tissue is noncompliant.[7] Another factor that puts the upper limb at risk for neuropathic pain is that few parts of the body are as mobile, or have the degree of excursion, as the nerves traveling from the cervical spine to the fingertips. These nerves cross multiple joint lines but, after

trauma, nerves can become tethered in immobile cutaneous scars surrounded by keratinocytes secreting chemokines and growth factors that promote painful neuromas.[8-13] Beyond the physical characteristics of the upper limb, many central and peripheral mechanisms also likely contribute to the development of chronic pain and undermine the results of a technically perfect surgery.[14]

Many physicians think that neuropathic pain is tingling or electrical and therefore complaints of sore, heavy, dull, or throbbing pain are considered not neuropathic in nature. However, surveys of patients with neuropathic pain, such as spinal cord injury pain, acute herpes zoster, postherpetic neuralgia, and diabetic neuropathy, found that this pain was often described as a dull throbbing or heavy pain.[15-20] Therefore the most important point in better treating the chronic pain after surgery is to recognize that this pain is more frequently than expected neuropathic in origin. There are some data suggesting that some of the medications that are frequently used to treat neuropathic pain work best for those people whose pain is not described in classic neuropathic

Department of Anesthesiology, Stanford University School of Medicine, Stanford Medicine Outpatient Center, Suite C-462, 450 Broadway Street, Redwood City, CA 94063, USA
E-mail address: irc39@pain.stanford.edu

Hand Clin 32 (2016) 51–61
http://dx.doi.org/10.1016/j.hcl.2015.08.011
0749-0712/16/$ – see front matter © 2016 Elsevier Inc. All rights reserved.

terms but who describe their pain as sore, dull, or heavy.[17–19]

Similarly, it is my own personal experience that cutaneous scar neuromas are invariably described by patients as a diffuse and deep pain. Therefore, no patient with chronic postsurgical pain can dissuade me from injecting their cutaneous scar with local anesthetic. For me, the only convincing evidence that a scar neuroma is not present and a major source of the patient's chronic pain is failure to have temporary profound analgesia in response to a scar injection with local anesthetic. Scar neuroma is an underexplored and underreported area of investigation in the literature on chronic postsurgical pain.

This article describes the basics of pharmacologic treatment of neuropathic pain (the most common type of chronic pain after surgery). This article is intended for upper extremity surgeons and allied practitioners who are not pain specialist but for whom a better understanding of how to treat nerve pain will be of great benefit.

GENERAL TENETS

1. Do not be in a hurry. The medications that most successfully reduce neuropathic pain and have the most durable analgesic effects all require some patience to be maximally successful. An expectation that they will work as quickly as commonly used pain relievers (opioid medications: eg, Vicodin, codeine) results in profound disappointment for both provider and patient. More importantly, impatience may cause you and your patient to prematurely put aside one of the few medications that can produce long-term profound pain relief. An expectation that neuropathic pain medicines will work on the time scales patients have come to expect from their previous exposure to opioids will cause a drug that might have been successful to be rejected. In addition to differing in their time to effectiveness, medications used for neuropathic chronic postsurgical pain also seem to have a threshold effect not commonly seen with the opioids. A patient may take a small quantity of an opioid and experience minor relief and know from experience that if they take more it is likely to provide greater relief. In contrast, many of the antidepressants and anticonvulsants used to manage neuropathic pain (henceforth referred to as antineuropathics) seem to have a threshold effect; a patient might feel no relief at 25 mg or 50 mg of nortriptyline, and then at 75 mg start to feel relief, and then at 150 mg feel profound relief. Patients' initial experience of the drug may therefore not reflect their subsequent experience with a higher dose.

2. Antineuropathics should be started at ineffective doses. When started at an effective doses antineuropathic medications often create side effects. These side effects can largely be avoided by slow titration from a low dose, which allows patients to accommodate to the medication effects. For example, duloxetine creates nausea in as many as 25% of patients when started an effective dose of 60 mg. However, if started at the ineffective dose of 20 mg a day, and then increasing the dose by 20 mg weekly up to 60 mg, then nausea becomes an infrequent side effect.[21–23] It is generally difficult to talk someone into retrying a drug that they are convinced makes them vomit (or be dopey and so forth), so it is better to start at a low, explicitly ineffective dose and gradually titrate up to an effective dose. I tell patients that I am going to give them a certain drug at a dose that does not work. We use the first few weeks not to help with the pain but just to get the patient's body used to this medication, then after a few weeks we start to explore doses that might help. Failure to have this kind of conversation with the patient results in loss of confidence in the physician and the medication when the medication fails to improve pain in the first few days.

3. There is some evidence that even though these drugs may exert some effect immediately at any given dose, the degree of pain relief may build substantially over the first few weeks of treatment.[22,23]

4. Unlike penicillin, for which there is a clear correct dose, with all of these antineuropathic medications doses have to be tailored to the individual. Given current technology it is impossible to know what dose may be too much for one person and not enough for another. Thus you have to test a given dose in a given person and then slowly change the dose to see the degree of side effects and the degree of pain relief. So the policy is:
   a. Start low (start at a dose that you are confident will not create side effects; usually a dose too low to be effective)
   b. Go slow (increase the dose by small increments every few days or each week so that you plan to reach the target dose in 1 to 2 months)
   c. But go! (when you start one of these medications do not just pick a low dose and leave it there, or decide that it does not work just because it is not having an effect at that low dose)

These medications should generally be slowly titrated up until:

i. The patient is getting significant pain relief, or

ii. The patient is reaching a dose defined by the medical literature to include some risk of sudden significant hazard (eg, desipramine at >200 mg/day is feared to cause an arrhythmia), or

iii. The patient is having dose-limiting side effects (eg, gabapentin is making a patient feel too sleepy or too nauseated)

5. Invest a small amount of effort into obtaining or making some dose titration schedules. It is cumbersome to write out dose titration schedules and this prevents people from gradually escalating the dose of medications (**Tables 1 and 2**). When clinicians write prescriptions like this: "Desipramine 25 mg; 1 to 6 tabs po qam; start 1 tab and increase according to dose schedule until taking 6 tabs po qam; dispense 180; 3 refills" they markedly reduce the problem of having the pharmacy dispense too few pills or having the insurance company cover too few pills.

6. Only change 1 thing at a time. People in pain want to get out of pain immediately and clinicians can be tempted to try multiple things at the same time. I am convinced that this strategy is always wrong. With this strategy, when the patient experiences side effects, neither patient nor physician knows which intervention is causing the side effect. Equally importantly, if intervention works, neither patient nor physician knows what is working. In both settings, patient and physician rely on previous beliefs about the medications and interventions to explain the results, resulting in a confirmation bias that may reinforce incorrect beliefs. For both physicians and patients, slowly learning what works and what does not, and why things do not work (eg, lack of efficacy vs overwhelming side effects), is important to eventually achieving success. Perhaps more importantly, if a physician only changes 1 thing at a time and then sees the result, and that experience is repeated by 100 or 1000 patients, then that physician develops much more accurate clinical acumen. Thus, the one-thing-at-a-time approach is just as important for becoming a better physician over time as it is for helping patients learn what really works and what are the trade-offs for that analgesia.

7. Make the patient commit to the process. In general, taking these medications one day

---

Table 1
Dosing schedule for desipramine (Norpramin 25 mg; also available as 10, 50, 75, 100, and 150 mg)

Week 1							
Day number	1	2	3	4	5	6	7
Morning	1	1	1	1	1	1	1
Week 2							
Day number	8	9	10	11	12	13	14
Morning	2	2	2	2	2	2	2
Week 3							
Day number	15	16	17	18	19	20	21
Morning	3	3	3	3	3	3	4
Week 4							
Day number	22	23	24	25	26	27	28
Morning	4	4	4	4	5	5	5
Week 5							
Day number	29	30	31	32	33	34	35[a]
Morning	5	5	5	6	6	6	6

#180 tablets dispersed (at 6 tabs by mouth every day).

If complete pain relief occurs, continue at that dose without further increases and call the pain clinic.

If concerning side effects occur, return to previous dose and call the pain clinic. Most side effects resolve with time, at which point the dose can again be escalated.

Potential side effects: dizziness, somnolence, fatigue, nausea, difficulty urinating, constipation, sexual dysfunction, arrhythmias, dry mouth, blurred vision, increased eye pressure in glaucoma, rash.

[a] Continue 6 tablets a day and call pain clinic to report results. We often do not see results until doses of 60 to 100 mg have been reached. Maximum initial dose is 150 mg/d.

Table 2
Dosing schedule for gabapentin (Neurontin 300 mg)

Week 1

Day number	1	2	3	4	5	6	7
Morning	0	0	0	1	1	1	1
Noon	0	0	0	0	0	0	0
Evening	1	1	1	1	1	1	1

Week 2

Day number	8	9	10	11	12	13	14
Morning	1	1	1	1	1	1	1
Noon	1	1	1	1	1	1	1
Evening	1	1	1	1	1	1	1

Week 3

Day number	15	16	17	18	19	20	21
Morning	1	1	1	1	1	1	1
Noon	1	1	1	2	2	2	2
Evening	2	2	2	2	2	2	2

Week 4

Day number	22	23	24	25	26	28	28
Morning	2	2	2	2	2	2	2
Noon	2	2	2	2	2	2	2
Evening	2	2	2	3	3	3	3

Week 5

Day number	29	30	31	32	33	34	35
Morning	2	2	2	2	3	3	3
Noon	3	3	3	3	3	3	3
Evening	3	3	3	3	3	3	3

Week 6

Day number	36	37	38	39	40	41	42
Morning	3	3	3	3	3	3	4
Noon	3	3	4	4	4	4	4
Evening	4	4	4	4	4	4	4

#360 tablets dispersed (at 4 tablets by mouth 3 times a day).

Potential side effects: dizziness, somnolence, fatigue, gastrointestinal upset, ataxia, tremor, abnormal vision or gait, abdominal pain, nystagmus, rash, headache, cognitive effect.

If during the increasing dosing schedule the patient develops any of these side effects, the patient should stop increasing the dose of medicine.

If the medicine has been providing pain relief, return to the dose that was taken before the occurrence of side effects.

and skipping them the next because of frustration makes the patient feel awful, so patients should commit to giving the medication a 6-week trial, or decide that they are not ready. The anticonvulsants and antidepressants used for nerve pain do not work when used haphazardly and patients become falsely educated that these medications do not work when in reality they are not working because of incorrect administration.

Neuropathic pain is a chronic condition that cannot always be fixed, and it is therefore important to introduce early the concept that neuropathic pain represents a chronic condition, like increased blood pressure, diabetes, or asthma, that requires long-term management rather than a fix. This message can be difficult to deliver, especially if the provider is the one who was operating at the time the chronic postsurgical pain began. Surgeons need to feel comfortable with the idea that the pain was caused by the surgery but it is almost certainly not the fault of the surgeon's technique or patient selection. Acceptance of the chronic disease paradigm at the initiation of treatment helps create a shared sense of realistic goals of treatment. I find it helpful to tell patients specifically which nerve is injured and that I cannot make the nerve the way it was before surgery. Every surgery cuts nerves because there are nerves in every part of the skin. In addition, I counsel that it is not known why most people only develop an area of numbness after surgery but a minority of patients develops nerve pain. I then reassure them that although I cannot fix their problem, I can help them have substantially less pain at the expense of having to take medications indefinitely (as for high blood pressure).

In addition, because chronic pain is also associated with depression and anxiety,[24] it is important that comorbid psychological disorders be treated aggressively. For this reason, it is often preferable to initiate treatment of neuropathic pain with a medication that addresses both pain and comorbid depression and anxiety. There are several agents that have activity in both the pain and psychological realms, including the tricyclic antidepressants (TCAs) and duloxetine.

There are few direct head-to-head trials of medications commonly used to treat neuropathic pain that would help specifically guide choice of one particular agent by efficacy. Among antidepressant drugs used for neuropathic pain the choice is between duloxetine (marketed as an extended release formulation under the brand name Cymbalta in the United States and more recently as a generic extended-release formulation as well) and the TCAs (amitriptyline, nortriptyline, and desipramine). The TCAs have been evaluated as treatments for neuropathic pain associated with diabetic neuropathy and postherpetic neuralgia in trials that often used a crossover design, and had sample sizes considerably smaller than more recent randomized controlled trials of duloxetine and pregabalin. To try to compare interventions, the Canadian Pain Society and others have used data based on number needed to treat (NNT) to compare different agents used for nerve pain.[25,26] The estimated NNT for the tricyclics in neuropathic pain is between 2 and 3. In contrast, the NNT for duloxetine based on duloxetine's 3 randomized controlled trials in diabetic neuropathy is closer to 5.[26] Other systematic reviews of the literature comparing the effectiveness of TCAs with that of gabapentin suggest the superiority of TCAs for treating neuropathic pain.[27]

TRICYCLIC ANTIDEPRESSANTS

TCAs were the first medications that proved effective for neuropathic pain in placebo-controlled trials. More than 17 placebo-controlled trials have shown the efficacy of TCAs for the treatment of neuropathic pain. The NNT for the TCAs is close to 2, suggesting a higher percentage of people may respond to TCAs than other medications. The primary problem with the use of TCAs is their adverse effect profile. TCAs must be used cautiously in patients with a history of cardiovascular disease, glaucoma, urinary retention, and the elderly. TCAs are not appropriate for patients at risk of overdose because of their well-described lethality in overdose. TCAs should also generally be avoided in patients currently being treated with selective serotonin reuptake inhibitors (SSRIs), for both pharmacokinetic and pharmacodynamic reasons. SSRIs inhibit the cytochrome P450 2D6 enzyme, which normally breaks down TCAs. Thus people taking SSRIs and TCAs at the same time are at risk of having marked increases in their TCA levels. Furthermore, the shared serotonin reuptake inhibition puts patients at risk of serotonin syndrome. Despite this, in rare monitored settings, the concurrent use of these medications can sometimes be accomplished safely.

Nortriptyline and desipramine are two of the tricyclics with the lowest affinity for the muscarinic cholinergic and histaminic receptors, and they therefore cause less sedation, constipation, and dry mouth than the more commonly prescribed amitriptyline (Elavil).[25,26,28] Desipramine in particular has the greatest noradrenergic profile and least antimuscarinic and antihistaminic profile of all the drugs in this class, making it particularly attractive among tricyclics.[28] Desipramine is usually slightly activating rather than sedating, and, in contrast with nortriptyline, is therefore better given in the morning than at night. Occasionally desipramine leads to difficulty sleeping because of its activating properties. However, perhaps because of its activating properties or its lower antihistaminic and anticholinergic profiles, desipramine does not seem to cause the same problematic weight gain seen with nortriptyline or amitriptyline. In contrast, nortriptyline is mildly sedating and is therefore better given at night.

Patients and practitioners must understand that TCAs have analgesic effects independent of their antidepressant effects. They are effective for relieving pain in people who are not depressed, they occasionally work for pain at doses that are not high enough to treat depression, and they work on time scales much faster for pain than for depression. TCAs such as desipramine should be initiated at a low dose (10–25 mg as a single dose) and then titrated every 3 to 7 days by 10 to 25 mg/day as tolerated. Although the analgesic effect of TCAs has been thought to occur at lower dosages than the antidepressant effects, there is evidence that higher doses of TCAs are markedly more effective than lower doses for the treatment of neuropathic pain.[29–31] TCAs should generally be titrated to dosages between 75 mg and 200 mg a day to maximize the likelihood of a good response. To ensure safety and to monitor for toxicity, electrocardiograms and blood levels should be checked once a patient reaches 150 mg/day. Blood levels of 500 ng/mL or higher are more likely to be associated with toxicity, with toxicity becoming the likely outcome of blood levels greater than 900 ng/mL. We typically target plasma concentrations between 100 and 300 ng/mL. Monitoring for toxicity is particularly important for desipramine. Desipramine may be the best-tolerated TCA, but, because of its potency, desipramine may also be particularly dangerous when given to patients with cardiac disease, or when taken in an overdose. Drug level monitoring identifies the patients with undesirably high or low plasma levels for appropriate action.[31]

Different individuals metabolize these medications differently because people can have different activity at the cytochrome P450 2D6 enzyme, the enzyme primarily responsible for digesting TCAs in the liver. Approximately 10% of caucasian have very limited activity at this enzyme, whereas between 20% and 30% of African Americans lack activity at this enzyme. Consequently these individuals with low activity can have very high blood levels when given normal doses of TCAs. In contrast, there is a smaller subset of individuals who are very rapid metabolizers. In these individuals, seemingly appropriate doses yield low blood levels that are ineffective, and following blood levels allows these patients to be identified and targeted for higher doses of TCA treatment.

In elderly patients TCAs may cause balance problems and cognitive impairment. Other adverse effects of TCAs include sedation, dry mouth, constipation, orthostasis, and occasionally weight gain. Weight gain best correlates with antihistaminic properties of the TCAs. Desipramine has markedly lower antihistaminic properties than other TCAs and does not seem to be associated with much, if any, weight gain; a notable problem with amitriptyline and nortriptyline.[28]

In addition to the higher efficacy of TCAs compared with other agents for neuropathic pain, other reasons to prefer initial treatment of neuropathic pain with TCAs include:

1. Their low cost.
2. Their effectiveness in treating comorbid depression. Comorbid depression occurs in up to 60% of individuals with chronic pain.

3. Once-a-day dosing with a half-life of approximately 23 hours improves ease of use and patient compliance, and therefore efficacy.
4. The ability to measure serum plasma levels and therefore identify patients who might otherwise fail treatment for pharmacokinetic reasons.
5. The wide range of doses available, from 10 mg to 300 mg as a single pill.
6. The reduced likelihood of causing cognitive side effects compared with anticonvulsant medications.

DULOXETINE AND VENLAFAXINE

Duloxetine and venlafaxine are selective norepinephrine and serotonin reuptake inhibitors (SNRIs). They therefore share some mechanistic similarities with TCAs, but lack the TCAs blockade of sodium channels and antagonism at alpha1-adrenergic, muscarinic cholinergic, and type 1 histamine receptors. The evidence for SNRI efficacy for neuropathic pain is much better established for duloxetine than for venlafaxine, which has shown mixed results and is not US Food and Drug Administration (FDA) approved for a pain indication, although we have seen patients respond to both.[22,23] Duloxetine is approved by the FDA to treat the pain associated with diabetic neuropathy. As described earlier, the NNT for duloxetine is perhaps twice as high as for the TCAs,[26] but duloxetine lacks the cardiac toxicity described for TCAs. We have found that duloxetine is noticeably less effective than TCAs. However, it may be well tolerated by some patients who are even worse candidates for TCAs or gabapentinoids; for example, the elderly. Some elderly patients develop clinically significant orthostatic hypertension with effective doses of duloxetine. Until recently it was only available as the branded drug Cymbalta, but now it is available as a generic sustained-release capsule. When started at a dose effective for nerve pain (60 mg or more) duloxetine causes nausea in at least one-quarter of patients.[22,32] However, this is easily avoided for most patients by starting at 20 mg/day and gradually escalating the dose to between 60 mg and 120 mg. Cases of fulminant hepatic failure have been reported for duloxetine and its use in patients with hepatic impairment is not recommended.[33] Patients who abruptly discontinue duloxetine or venlafaxine after spending several months on either medication may become very unhappy and report a variety of bizarre somatic and cognitive symptoms, as well as emotional lability and extreme feelings of despondence.[34,35] Several of our patients have described feeling electrical zaps throughout their bodies on sudden cessation of duloxetine. These symptoms have been reported by others as well.[36] These symptoms stop abruptly on reinitiating duloxetine, but may persist for weeks if the patient decides to persist rather than reinitiate the duloxetine.

GABAPENTINOIDS

Gabapentin and pregabalin (collectively termed gabapentinoids) should be considered first-line treatment of neuropathic pain. These medications have a shared mechanism of action, which seems to involve the modulation of voltage-gated calcium channels existing on presynaptic pain-carrying neurons in the dorsal horn of the spinal cord. It is thought that the action of gabapentin and pregabalin on these voltage-gated calcium channels inhibits the presynaptic release of pronociceptive neurotransmitters such as glutamate and nociceptive peptides.[37] These medications have proven efficacy for the treatment of neuropathic pain arising from diabetic peripheral neuropathy[38–41] and postherpetic neuralgia.[42–45] Their use in chronic postsurgical pain stems from an appreciation that chronic postsurgical pain often arises from nerve injury. Studies suggest that the NNT for these medications ranges from 4 to 6.5.[26]

The structure of gabapentin is similar to that of an amino acid and, unlike many medications, gabapentin relies on an active transport process for absorption, a process that can be saturated.[46] Consequently the absorption of gabapentin from the duodenum is nonlinear, with progressively lower increments of gabapentin being absorbed is the dose increases. This property provides gabapentin with both a built-in safety mechanism and also a built-in efficacy ceiling because patients can only absorb so much gabapentin at a time. Consequently, to become overmedicated with gabapentin usually requires either some impairment that makes the patient unusually susceptible to the effects of cognitively impairing medications, or alternatively the patient has to have a defect in gabapentin elimination. Gabapentin is normally excreted unchanged by the kidneys so gabapentin can accumulate in patients with renal insufficiency,[47] causing significant cognitive impairment, oversedation, and myoclonus.[48]

Pregabalin (Lyrica) has the same mechanism of action as gabapentin[49] but differs primarily in the pharmacokinetics governing its absorption from the intestines. Pregabalin is not dependent on an active transport process in the duodenum that can be saturated, but is absorbed more diffusely throughout the intestines and has linear pharmacokinetics at clinically relevant doses in humans. Because it has a shared molecular mechanism of

action with gabapentin, it is hard to explain the occasional patients who report that they tolerate pregabalin but experienced cognitive side effects with gabapentin. Nonetheless, as a general rule, pregabalin should not be the first drug trialed among patients reporting cognitive side effects from gabapentin, because a better-absorbed version of a drug with the same mechanism of action should not be relied on to result in fewer side effects. However, for that subgroup of patients who are inclined to take a higher dose of gabapentin because of inadequate analgesia, and the absence of dose-limiting side effects, but are unlikely to be able to absorb higher doses of gabapentin (ie, they are taking a dose close to the maximum absorbable amount; roughly 3600 mg/day), switching to pregabalin, or alternatively augmenting with pregabalin, may bypass the dose-limiting bottleneck presented by inadequate duodenal absorption of gabapentin.

COMBINATIONS

There are several high-quality studies of medication combinations for neuropathic pain, but few of the combinations have been replicated. The exception to this is the combination of an opioid plus gabapentin. A recent meta-analysis of 386 subjects from 2 trials showed statistically significant but clinically modest superiority of gabapentin when combined with an opioid compared with gabapentin alone.[50]

A well-done but small study of the combination of nortriptyline and gabapentin evaluated either drug versus the combination of both drugs.[51] The study was a double-blind, double-dummy, crossover trial of patients with neuropathic pain who were randomized in a 1:1:1 ratio to gabapentin, nortriptyline, or the combination. Each group was then crossed over to experience each of the other 2 groups. Overall the combination was statistically significantly more effective than either drug alone. This finding in the setting of a small sample size suggests an effect size that is large and that is likely to be clinically meaningful as well. Our own experience is in agreement with these findings. In addition, although these results were obtained in patients with either diabetic neuropathy or postherpetic neuralgia, our own experience suggests that the same agents and combinations seem to be effective in the setting of neuropathic pain caused by postsurgical traumatic nerve injury. In practice, most patients benefit from a combination of medications but the scientific basis of this approach remains limited, with few data to suggest improved efficacy or reduced side effects.

OPIOIDS

Several different opioids have been examined in randomized controlled trials for the treatment of neuropathic pain conditions, including painful diabetic neuropathy, postherpetic neuralgia, sciatica, postamputation pain, and spinal cord injury pain.[25] Overall, these trials seem to support the belief that opioids confer a moderate improvement in pain as well as an improvement in function in patients with neuropathic pain. However, most of the studies are limited by having a short duration. This limitation is particularly problematic because, unlike the antidepressants and anticonvulsants, opioid use results in a greater degree of tolerance, so although it is clear that opioids are helpful when first initiated for neuropathic pain, it is less clear that opioids remain effective for neuropathic pain over time. Furthermore, the adverse side effects of opioids, and in particular the increasing levels of prescription opioid misuse that has paralleled the increased availability of prescription opioids, have left many prescribers wondering whether the benefits are worth the costs.

LAMOTRIGINE

Lamotrigine (Lamictal) has had positive results treating neuropathic pain related to human immunodeficiency virus–induced neuropathy, trigeminal neuralgia, and central pain. Two large clinical trials in diabetic neuropathy showed a nonsignificant trends toward a positive effect ($P = .07$).[52] Overall, the data suggest that lamotrigine may be helpful for some people with neuropathic pain but likely has an effect size smaller than that of the gabapentinoids, TCAs, and duloxetine. Lamotrigine is thought to reduce neuropathic pain through several mechanisms, including sodium channel blockade. In addition, lamotrigine has some serious issues that make it challenging for routine treatment. One in 10 people develops a rash,[53] most commonly in children, patients taking valproic acid or carbamazepine, and those increasing the dose of lamotrigine by more than 25 mg every 2 weeks.[54] The occurrence of this rash with more rapid dose escalation mandates a prolonged period of time between starting lamotrigine and achieving what can be an effective therapeutic dose (typically around 100 mg twice a day). Furthermore, roughly 1 in 1000 people develop a Stevens-Johnson–type syndrome, the potential for which necessitates the cessation of treatment during the occurrence of the much more common rash of a non–Stevens-Johnson type.[55] In contrast, lamotrigine is generally well tolerated with a lower incidence of significant weight gain

or cognitive dysfunction compared with gabapentin or pregabalin.

TOPIRAMATE

Topiramate is a second-generation antiepileptic medication that has shown significant efficacy in a variety of headache syndromes as well as in certain seizure disorders. It has several purported mechanisms of action, including sodium channel blockade, GABAergic effects, and carbonic anhydrase inhibition.[56] Early studies of topiramate seemed to show promise for neuropathic pain[57,58] and 1 large randomized controlled trial showed topiramate to be superior to placebo in reducing the pain among patients with painful diabetic peripheral neuropathy.[58] A follow-on open-label extension also seemed to support the efficacy and sustained pain relief of topiramate for neuropathic pain.[59] However, another group of 3 randomized controlled trials of topiramate for diabetic peripheral neuropathy failed to show a statistically significant effect for topiramate treatment.[60] These studies have been criticized for methodological flaws that might have contributed to a failure to find a real treatment effect of topiramate. These methodological flaws included enrollment of patients whose pain was not particularly severe with a possible floor effect; permission during the study for patients to use opioid analgesics as rescue medication; and a failure to specifically reference lower extremity pain when inquiring about pain and pain relief related to study medication. Note that in the large randomized, placebo-controlled trial that did find a clinically meaningful effect of topiramate to reduce neuropathic pain, these methodological issues were not involved.[58] This randomized, placebo-controlled, multicenter, 12-week study included 323 subjects with pain greater than a 4 out of 10 on a visual analog scale. Fifty percent of patients treated with topiramate experienced a clinically meaningful reduction in pain (defined as 30% or greater reduction in pain on a visual analog score) compared with 34% of placebo-treated subjects ($P = .004$). Topiramate also improved sleep and reduced worst pain intensity. Unlike most of the drugs that are used for nerve pain, topiramate seems to induce weight loss, and resulted in an average 2.6-kg weight loss over 12 weeks among patients with painful diabetic neuropathy. In our practice, few patients seem to have profound relief with Topamax. However, for the minority of patients who do achieve relief, the relief is often significant. Among these patients, the doses at which relief occurs tend to be in the higher dose ranges; often as high as 400 to 600 mg/day. In contrast, an open-label

26-week study to assess the long-term safety and effectiveness of topiramate among patients with painful diabetic peripheral neuropathy evaluated 205 subjects taking doses up to 600 mg/day and concluded that pain relief was effective and durable. This study suggested that as many as 40% of patients discontinue topiramate. Patients most frequently discontinue because of adverse effects, including cognitive impairment, sedation, lack of appetite, paresthesia, and gastrointestinal upset.[59] We have also rarely seen patients discontinue this medication despite efficacy because of progressive hair thinning. In addition, likely because of its carbonic anhydrase activity, topiramate is associated with an increased incidence of nephrolithiasis. Clinicians familiar with topiramate (marketed in the United States as Topamax) jokingly refer to it as Dopamax because of the sedation. Nonetheless, a small minority of patients seem to be impervious to the cognitive side effects of topiramate and tolerate it at fairly high doses with corresponding pain relief. Patient acceptance of topiramate is often high in the office when patients hear that it may induce weight loss, but enthusiasm wanes quickly when cognitive side effects occur. In addition, female patients should be advised that topiramate may reduce the effectiveness of oral contraceptive pills.[61]

TOPICAL MEDICATIONS
Lidocaine

Lidoderm is a 5% lidocaine patch that won approval based on its effectiveness in postherpetic neuralgia. It seems to work locally because systemic levels are negligible, and systemic side effects are virtually nonexistent. It was hoped that it would be effective in particular for people with cutaneous nerve injuries such as scar neuromas, a common affliction following upper extremity and hand surgery. However, our experience using topical lidocaine gels or the Lidoderm patch for topical treatment of postsurgical cutaneous nerve injuries has been generally disappointing. We have seen some rare patients who report the Lidoderm patch to be helpful, but these patients are the exception rather than the rule. Furthermore, it is often difficult to get Lidoderm patches covered for conditions other than postherpetic neuralgia. For this reason we often prescribe a small quantity of patches to patients with postsurgical cutaneous nerve injuries and inform patients that they have to pay for it themselves initially. We then try to get it approved for the much smaller number of patients who report to us that they find it useful. However, given the unique safety and virtual absence of systemic side effects, it is hard to argue against a trial of topical lidocaine in patients with cutaneous nerve injuries.

Capsaicin

Topical capsaicin, the active ingredient in hot chili peppers, seems to help some patients with postherpetic neuralgia. Although capsaicin initially causes increased pain by activating sensory nerve fibers in the skin, repeated persistent application of over-the-counter–strength capsaicin (less than 1%) causes desensitization and pain relief with some long-lasting but temporary regression of pain fibers from the skin. More recently, the approval of a high-dose capsaicin patch (8%) has allowed some patients to get persistent relief from a single application. There is at least 1 case report of complex regional pain syndrome (CRPS) symptoms getting worse following application of capsaicin patch. Therefore, use of the high-dose capsaicin patch in patients who have developed CRPS following hand surgery should be approached with caution.[62]

CONCLUSION

The treatment of pain is a complex process that requires a team approach. This article provides an overview of the pharmaceutical treatments available. One of the goals is to give providers treating upper extremity disorders more tools to treat their patients with chronic pain. Another goal is to improve hand providers' understanding of the medications their pain colleagues prescribe in shared patients. Pharmaceuticals are an important component in the treatment of chronic pain and opioids are often not a good solution. Knowing what other medications are available can improve the care for these challenging patients.

REFERENCES

1. Kehlet H, Jensen TS, Woolf CJ. Persistent postsurgical pain: risk factors and prevention. Lancet 2006;367(9522):1618–25.
2. Henderson J, Terenghi G, McGrouther DA, et al. The reinnervation pattern of wounds and scars may explain their sensory symptoms. J Plast Reconstr Aesthet Surg 2006;59(9):942–50.
3. Hazari A, Elliot D. Treatment of end-neuromas, neuromas-in-continuity and scarred nerves of the digits by proximal relocation. J Hand Surg Br 2004;29(4): 338–50.
4. Defalque RJ. Painful trigger points in surgical scars. Anesth Analg 1982;61(6):518–20.
5. White JC. The problem of the painful scar. Ann Surg 1958;148(3):422–32.

6. Masear VR. Nerve wrapping. Foot Ankle Clin 2011; 16(2):327–37.

7. Bouche P. Compression and entrapment neuropathies. Handb Clin Neurol 2013;115:311–66.

8. Birklein F, Drummond PD, Li W, et al. Activation of cutaneous immune responses in complex regional pain syndrome. J Pain 2014;15(5):485–95.

9. Peleshok JC, Ribeiro-da-Silva A. Neurotrophic factor changes in the rat thick skin following chronic constriction injury of the sciatic nerve. Mol Pain 2012;8:1.

10. Li WW, Guo TZ, Li XQ, et al. Fracture induces keratinocyte activation, proliferation, and expression of pro-nociceptive inflammatory mediators. Pain 2010; 151(3):843–52.

11. Dussor G, Koerber HR, Oaklander AL, et al. Nucleotide signaling and cutaneous mechanisms of pain transduction. Brain Res Rev 2009;60(1):24–35.

12. Curtin C, Carroll I. Cutaneous neuroma physiology and its relationship to chronic pain. J Hand Surg Am 2009;34(7):1334–6.

13. Guo TZ, Wei T, Li WW, et al. Immobilization contributes to exaggerated neuropeptide signaling, inflammatory changes, and nociceptive sensitization after fracture in rats. J Pain 2014;15(10):1033–45.

14. Wang CK, Myunghae Hah J, Carroll I. Factors contributing to pain chronicity. Curr Pain Headache Rep 2009;13(1):7–11.

15. Cepeda MS, Wilcox M, Levitan B. Pain qualities and satisfaction with therapy: a survey of subjects with neuropathic pain. Pain Med 2013;14(11):1745–56.

16. Celik EC, Erhan B, Lakse E. The clinical characteristics of neuropathic pain in patients with spinal cord injury. Spinal Cord 2012;50(8):585–9.

17. Mackey S, Carroll I, Emir B, et al. Sensory pain qualities in neuropathic pain. J Pain 2012;13(1):58–63.

18. Carroll IR, Younger JW, Mackey SC. Pain quality predicts lidocaine analgesia among patients with suspected neuropathic pain. Pain Med 2010;11(4): 617–21.

19. Gilron I, Tu D, Holden RR. Sensory and affective pain descriptors respond differentially to pharmacological interventions in neuropathic conditions. Clin J Pain 2013;29(2):124–31.

20. Loncar Z, Mestrovic AH, Bilic M, et al. Quality of pain in herpes zoster patients. Coll Antropol 2013;37(2): 527–30.

21. Castro-Diaz D, Palma PC, Bouchard C, et al. Effect of dose escalation on the tolerability and efficacy of duloxetine in the treatment of women with stress urinary incontinence. Int Urogynecol J Pelvic Floor Dysfunct 2007;18(8):919–29.

22. Goldstein DJ, Lu Y, Detke MJ, et al. Duloxetine vs. placebo in patients with painful diabetic neuropathy. Pain 2005;116(1–2):109–18.

23. Raskin J, Pritchett YL, Wang F, et al. A double-blind, randomized multicenter trial comparing duloxetine with placebo in the management of diabetic peripheral neuropathic pain. Pain Med 2005;6(5):346–56.

24. Bair MJ, Robinson RL, Katon W, et al. Depression and pain comorbidity: a literature review. Arch Intern Med 2003;163(20):2433–45.

25. Moulin D, Boulanger A, Clark AJ, et al. Pharmacological management of chronic neuropathic pain: revised consensus statement from the Canadian Pain Society. Pain Res Manag 2014;19(6):328–35.

26. Finnerup NB, Sindrup SH, Jensen TS. The evidence for pharmacological treatment of neuropathic pain. Pain 2010;150(3):573–81.

27. Chou R, Carson S, Chan BK. Gabapentin versus tricyclic antidepressants for diabetic neuropathy and postherpetic neuralgia: discrepancies between direct and indirect meta-analyses of randomized controlled trials. J Gen Intern Med 2009;24(2):178–88.

28. Gillman PK. Tricyclic antidepressant pharmacology and therapeutic drug interactions updated. Br J Pharmacol 2007;151(6):737–48.

29. Sindrup SH, Gram LF, Skjold T, et al. Clomipramine vs desipramine vs placebo in the treatment of diabetic neuropathy symptoms. A double-blind cross-over study. Br J Clin Pharmacol 1990;30(5): 683–91.

30. Sindrup SH, Gram LF, Skjold T, et al. Concentration-response relationship in imipramine treatment of diabetic neuropathy symptoms. Clin Pharmacol Ther 1990;47(4):509–15.

31. Rasmussen PV, Jensen TS, Sindrup SH, et al. TDM-based imipramine treatment in neuropathic pain. Ther Drug Monit 2004;26(4):352–60.

32. Greist J, McNamara RK, Mallinckrodt CH, et al. Incidence and duration of antidepressant-induced nausea: duloxetine compared with paroxetine and fluoxetine. Clin Ther 2004;26(9):1446–55.

33. Hanje AJ, Pell LJ, Votolato NA, et al. Case report: fulminant hepatic failure involving duloxetine hydrochloride. Clin Gastroenterol Hepatol 2006;4(7):912–7.

34. Perahia DG, Kajdasz DK, Desaiah D, et al. Symptoms following abrupt discontinuation of duloxetine treatment in patients with major depressive disorder. J Affect Disord 2005;89(1–3):207–12.

35. Hou YC, Lai CH. Long-term duloxetine withdrawal syndrome and management in a depressed patient. J Neuropsychiatry Clin Neurosci 2014;26(1):E4.

36. Pitchot W, Ansseau M. Shock-like sensations associated with duloxetine discontinuation. Ann Clin Psychiatry 2008;20(3):175.

37. Maneuf YP, Luo ZD, Lee K. $\alpha 2\delta$ and the mechanism of action of gabapentin in the treatment of pain. Semin Cell Dev Biol 2006;17(5):565–70.

38. Backonja M, Beydoun A, Edwards KR, et al. Gabapentin for the symptomatic treatment of painful neuropathy in patients with diabetes mellitus: a randomized controlled trial. JAMA 1998;280(21): 1831–6.

39. Backonja MM. Gabapentin monotherapy for the symptomatic treatment of painful neuropathy: a multicenter, double-blind, placebo-controlled trial in patients with diabetes mellitus. Epilepsia 1999; 40(Suppl 6):S57–9 [discussion: S73–4].

40. Lesser H, Sharma U, LaMoreaux L, et al. Pregabalin relieves symptoms of painful diabetic neuropathy: a randomized controlled trial. Neurology 2004;63(11): 2104–10.

41. Rosenstock J, Tuchman M, LaMoreaux L, et al. Pregabalin for the treatment of painful diabetic peripheral neuropathy: a double-blind, placebo-controlled trial. Pain 2004;110(3):628–38.

42. Sabatowski R, Galvez R, Cherry DA, et al. Pregabalin reduces pain and improves sleep and mood disturbances in patients with post-herpetic neuralgia: results of a randomised, placebo-controlled clinical trial. Pain 2004;109(1–2):26–35.

43. Dworkin RH, Corbin AE, Young JP Jr, et al. Pregabalin for the treatment of postherpetic neuralgia: a randomized, placebo-controlled trial. Neurology 2003; 60(8):1274–83.

44. Rice AS, Maton S, Postherpetic Neuralgia Study Group. Gabapentin in postherpetic neuralgia: a randomised, double blind, placebo controlled study. Pain 2001;94(2):215–24.

45. Rowbotham M, Harden N, Stacey B, et al. Gabapentin for the treatment of postherpetic neuralgia: a randomized controlled trial. JAMA 1998;280(21):1837–42.

46. Stewart BH, Kugler AR, Thompson PR, et al. A saturable transport mechanism in the intestinal absorption of gabapentin is the underlying cause of the lack of proportionality between increasing dose and drug levels in plasma. Pharm Res 1993; 10(2):276–81.

47. Wong MO, Eldon MA, Keane WF, et al. Disposition of gabapentin in anuric subjects on hemodialysis. J Clin Pharmacol 1995;35(6):622–6.

48. Kaufman KR, Parikh A, Chan L, et al. Myoclonus in renal failure: two cases of gabapentin toxicity. Epilepsy Behav Case Rep 2014;2:8–10.

49. Taylor CP, Angelotti T, Fauman E. Pharmacology and mechanism of action of pregabalin: the calcium channel alpha2-delta (alpha2 delta) subunit as a target for antiepileptic drug discovery. Epilepsy Res 2007;73(2):137–50.

50. Chaparro LE, Wiffen PJ, Moore RA, et al. Combination pharmacotherapy for the treatment of neuropathic pain in adults. Cochrane Database Syst Rev 2012;7:CD008943.

51. Gilron I, Bailey JM, Tu D, et al. Nortriptyline and gabapentin, alone and in combination for neuropathic pain: a double-blind, randomised controlled cross-over trial. Lancet 2009;374(9697):1252–61.

52. Vinik AI, Tuchman M, Safirstein B, et al. Lamotrigine for treatment of pain associated with diabetic neuropathy: results of two randomized, double-blind, placebo-controlled studies. Pain 2007;128(1–2): 169–79.

53. Wang XQ, Xiong J, Xu WH, et al. Risk of a lamotrigine-related skin rash: current meta-analysis and postmarketing cohort analysis. Seizure 2015; 25:52–61.

54. Hirsch LJ, Weintraub DB, Buchsbaum R, et al. Predictors of lamotrigine-associated rash. Epilepsia 2006;47(2):318–22.

55. Hussain N, Gosalakkal JA. Lamotrigine rash-a potentially life-threatening complication. BMJ Case Rep 2009;2009. bcr2006037754.

56. Shank RP, Gardocki JF, Streeter AJ, et al. An overview of the preclinical aspects of topiramate: pharmacology, pharmacokinetics, and mechanism of action. Epilepsia 2000;41(Suppl 1):S3–9.

57. Kline KM, Carroll DG, Malnar KF. Painful diabetic peripheral neuropathy relieved with use of oral topiramate. South Med J 2003;96(6):602–5.

58. Raskin P, Donofrio PD, Rosenthal NR, et al. Topiramate vs placebo in painful diabetic neuropathy: analgesic and metabolic effects. Neurology 2004; 63(5):865–73.

59. Donofrio PD, Raskin P, Rosenthal NR, et al. Safety and effectiveness of topiramate for the management of painful diabetic peripheral neuropathy in an open-label extension study. Clin Ther 2005;27(9):1420–31.

60. Thienel U, Neto W, Schwabe SK, et al, Topiramate Diabetic Neuropathic Pain Study Group. Topiramate in painful diabetic polyneuropathy: findings from three double-blind placebo-controlled trials. Acta Neurol Scand 2004;110(4):221–31.

61. Rosenfeld WE, Doose DR, Walker SA, et al. Effect of topiramate on the pharmacokinetics of an oral contraceptive containing norethindrone and ethinyl estradiol in patients with epilepsy. Epilepsia 1997; 38(3):317–23.

62. Girtler R, Kloimstein H, Gustorff B. Pronounced symptom deterioration in complex regional pain syndrome type II after isolated application of a highly concentrated capsaicin patch. A case report. Schmerz 2013;27(1):67–71 [in German].

Hand Therapy Treatment

Susan W. Stralka, PT, DPT, MS

KEYWORDS

- Pain • Mechanism of pain • Peripheral and central mechanisms • Upper quadrant evaluation
- Abnormal impulse generators • Mirror therapy and graded motor imagery

KEY POINTS

- Pain is a multifactorial process.
- Treatment must target all pain mechanisms.
- Specific treatments include upper limb neurodynamic therapy.
- Specific treatments include mirror therapy and graded motor imagery.
- Treatment of pain must be holistic including the peripheral and central nervous system.

INTRODUCTION

Treating pain is a common part of the therapist's daily routine. Therapists dealing with upper extremity pain often look for the peripheral symptoms and design a treatment program solely aimed at treating the peripheral symptoms. We have all been taught that pain is a normal physiologic response that provides a survival advantage to our bodies. Pain from tissue damage triggers protective behaviors preventing further damage and allowing for the healing and repair processes to occur. Pain serves as a warning sign to alert an individual of potential harm so that an appropriate response can result.[1] However, this protective response does not represent a complete picture of pain. Pain can morph from a healthy protection to a pathologic response that prevents recovery.

Pain is a complex process propagated by many systems: the level of injury, the peripheral nervous system, and the central nervous system (CNS). Thus, therapists treating hand injuries must consider pain using a broad holistic perspective. One must assess the damaged tissue with its peripheral pain symptoms but also consider that there may be a CNS component contributing to the pain. With pain and persistent pain (pain continuing after the tissue has healed), it is the brain that makes a decision if the input is dangerous and if so what action to take. The CNS, brain, and spinal cord can become sensitive to a nociceptive input resulting in more pain with less provocation. It is important to realize that the brain not only responds to physical stimuli but also inputs from thoughts and emotions.

This article covers recent advancements in the neuroscience of pain that impact evolving strategies to identify and treat pain mechanisms. The use of physical agents for upper extremity musculoskeletal pain management is not the focus of this article, but is found in the literature.[2] We discuss recent research focused on pain mechanisms, which has highlighted the importance of pain behaviors and afforded evidence in the most effective treatment strategies for better functional outcomes.

IMPORTANCE OF PAIN

Pain is often the reason patients seek medical care. For the upper limb, pain can be extremely debilitating, impacting many basic daily functions. According to Butler,[3] pain is a complex unique experience to each individual: there is no pain exactly alike. The International Association for Study of Pain has helped define the terminology of pain. The International Association for Study of Pain defines pain as an unpleasant sensory and emotional experience associated with actual or potential tissue damage. Pain is multidimensional, involving not only the sensation of pain but also the

3033 Poplar Grove Lane, Germantown, TN 38139, USA
E-mail address: susanwstralka@bellsouth.net

Hand Clin 32 (2016) 63–69
http://dx.doi.org/10.1016/j.hcl.2015.08.007
0749-0712/16/$ – see front matter © 2016 Elsevier Inc. All rights reserved.

emotional experience with which it is associated. The International Association for Study of Pain also suggested that pain should be categorized in terms of the mechanisms causing the pain, not by a time factor, such as acute and chronic.[4,5]

One of the challenges for clinicians treating pain is to move past the sole focus on the injured tissue. A not uncommon clinical scenario is the physician frustrated with a patient whose bone is healed but is still complaining of pain. According to Woolf,[4] health care providers continue to believe that pain in the absence of tissue pathology is not real. Unfortunately, there is a lack understanding of the "neurobiologic phenomenon" that generated pain without obvious noxious stimuli. The pain in these patients is not always caused by secondary gains (work, or insurance-related compensation), opioid drug seeking, and psychiatric disturbances (ie, malingering, lying, or hysterics). Therapists can serve a critical role in treating the patient at every level including the pain generated from central mechanisms.

In the past, acute pain has been described as a direct result of tissue damage in which free nerve endings called nociceptors (sensory neurons) are activated by noxious stimuli. In the hand, the nociceptors are located in the skin, muscles, tendons, boney structures, and within the nervi nervorum in peripheral nerves. Historically clinicians have most commonly treated the nociceptive input. This was appropriate when the pain mechanisms were nociceptive in nature, such as the pain immediately following injury or postoperatively. However, what is the correct clinical strategy for treating a patient that has allodynia (nonpainful stimuli that is painful) and is hypersensitive (an increased response to a stimuli that is normally painful)? These patients will not move their limb because of the fear of moving or the misunderstanding that movement is harmful. This is where one must identify and treat other pain mechanisms (central and/or peripheral) on the initial assessment before initiating a treatment plan. The treatment modalities differ depending on what is generating the pain.

The three main categories of pain generators are (1) peripheral nociceptive, (2) peripheral neurogenic, and (3) central sensitization. Central sensitization is an area of increasing focus. It is thought to be the site accountable for the maintenance of persistent pain that cannot be explained by peripheral tissue damage. It is also thought to play a large role in chronic pain. According to Sluka,[6] pain is considered chronic if the pain lasts more than normal tissue healing time, the impairment is greater than expected, and the symptoms now occurring may not be from identifiable tissue damage. Reviewed next are the mechanism for the three categories of pain.

PAIN MECHANISMS
Peripheral Nociceptive

Peripheral nocioceptive pain results from peripheral tissue damage or potential tissue damage. This is often the acute pain commonly seen after trauma and is a symptom of the tissue injury. Therapists are comfortable treating peripheral nociceptive pain. They can identify hand tissue damage from trauma, overuse, or surgery. Peripheral nociceptive pain symptoms are from a clear pathology and have a predictable time frame to get better, which is usually within 3 months.

Peripheral nociceptive pain is generated by various traumas, such as chemical, mechanical, or thermal injury. The acute response to noxious insults produces an inflammatory response that begins the process of healing. These responses include peripheral impulse generators carried by specific sensory receptors called nociceptors. With peripheral nociceptive input the course of the injury usually follows a predictable pattern and the symptoms decrease because there is a reduction in inflammation as healing occurs.

Patients with nociceptive and inflammatory pain complain of intermittent sharp pain with movement; constant dull ache or throb at rest, localized to the areas of injury; and clear, proportionate mechanical and anatomic in nature to aggravating and easing factors. Hand therapist intervention is most helpful for pain management and tissue healing during the time frame of the peripheral nociceptive mechanisms. The usual therapy interventions include patient education, pain management, and treatment of edema, protection of the joints by orthoses, range of motion, and the progression of normal movement patterns, and activities of daily living.

Peripheral Neurogenic

The peripheral neurogenic mechanism moves beyond the tissue that was directly injured. Peripheral neurogenic pain is related to activation of nerves anywhere from the exit of the spinal cord to the distal segments of the peripheral nervous system. This category includes neuropathic pain, but is not specifically discussed. Peripheral neurogenic pain symptoms may be generated anywhere along the course of the nerve from a cervical radicular neuropathy to a distal branch of a nerve. Peripheral neurogenic pain can present a challenge to the clinician because distal nerve injury signs and symptoms may originate from a more proximal nerve injury.

Neurogenic pain originates from neural tissue outside the dorsal horn of the spinal cord and includes nerve root symptoms, peripheral nerve entrapment, and pain associated with neuroma.[7] Untreated inflammation surrounding a nerve can contribute to the pain process. Edema and inflammation can increase pressure on nerves. Repetitive compressive, friction, vibration, and anatomically narrow tissue spaces through which the neural structures pass often cause mechanical irritation. Each peripheral nerve is one cell extending from the spinal cord to its end organ. If any part of the nerve is injured, the entire nerve becomes more susceptible to injury. This phenomenon is called double crush syndrome, named by Upton and McComas in 1973.[8] Double crush means that multiple sites of one nerve may be responsible for the pain. Thus, the clinician must be aware and treat all entrapment sites to allow for recovery and pain relief.

The symptom pattern for peripheral neurogenic pain usually is painful sensation with pins and needles, burning for a superficial nerve, or cramping sensation for deeper nerve. Pain is usually evoked by movement of a nerve related to pressure gradient changes around that nerve. Patients have described their pain as "wires are pulling on my nerves," "fire ants are crawling up my nerve then stinging me," or "my arm feels as if hot wax is dripping down it." It is not uncommon to see musculoskeletal conditions, such as tennis elbow, carpal tunnel syndrome, de Quervain disease, and whiplash, also resulting in peripheral nerve irritation. Patients have changes in perception; lower threshold to stimuli; and proprioceptive deficits including errors in repositioning, decreased position sense, and difficulty adopting postures as seen in a picture or photograph. Sensory alterations include stimuli being processed more slowly, incorrect localization, and decreased accuracy in recognition of tactile stimuli. Patients with neurogenic pain may have a history of other nerve injury. Neurogenic pain usually follows a dermatome or cutaneous distribution, whereas symptoms are provoked by tension or load on neural tissue causing numbness, paresthesias, or muscle weakness. A patient may have both nociceptive and neurogenic symptoms after traumatic injuries. The physical examination signs of nociceptive pain following tissue damage consist of stiffness, redness, and warmth often related to the normal inflammatory process following injury. The peripheral neurogenic clinical signs consist of numbness, tingling, and burning associated with tension on a nerve.

Examination should include a full upper quadrant evaluation from spinal foramen to fingertip to identify and differentiate peripheral neurogenic signs from nociceptive signs. Upper quadrant evaluation should identify the primary sources of musculoskeletal weakness and pain symptoms causing the impairment. The underlying mechanisms for most therapy interventions to decrease pain are based on reducing the inflammatory response in healing tissue, modulating pain via the gating mechanisms and releasing endogenous opioids, restoring muscle function, and moving a nerve.[2]

What if the patient with presumed peripheral neurogenic pain does not respond to peripheral treatment of splinting, edema reduction, joint and tendon mobilization, nerve gliding, strengthening, and ergonomic intervention? Consider that the CNS may be a component of the pain process and implement appropriate treatments (these are described in more detail later).

Central Pain or Central Sensitization

Central pain or central sensitization is the third mechanism contributing to pain. Central pain results from dysfunction of the CNS. Woolf[4] stated that peripheral nociceptive input into the CNS pathways can trigger prolonged but reversible increased neuronal excitability and decreased inhibitory influences. Neuroplastic changes within different areas of the CNS may help to explain the transition from acute to chronic conditions and peripheral nociceptive conditions to central sensitization. Clinically, central pain can present to providers as a puzzling array of symptoms. Patients with central sensitization can have sensory-motor dysfunction, perceptual disturbances, and disproportional and persistent pain with no structural cause.[9] Also, this pain can spread to other body areas. At the central level, both the facilitory and inhibitory pain pathways can be modulated by the injury, anxiety, attention to the pain, and stress.[10] Clinicians often see patients who have their symptoms spread around the body; pain is out of proportion; abnormal sensations, such as allodynia and hyperalgesia (painful sensation is magnified and can spread); along with unusual movements, such as focal dystonia. Patients often state that their hand or upper extremity is sensitive to any material touching it and even thinking about moving the limb is painful. It has been proposed that persistent pain associated with musculoskeletal disorders is a result of imprinting a learned response that has formed a maladaptive memory sustaining the chronic pain.[11] The CNS is where the psychological and physiologic factors become intertwined. If central sensitization is suspected exercises to retrain the brain should start immediately targeting the physical and the psychological aspects to improve the outcome.[12]

Persistent pain results in structural changes in the brain. These changes include decreased gray matter, reorganization of motor and sensory areas in the brain, and abnormal connectivity within the brain.[13–15] Nijs and colleagues[16] describe central sensitivity in musculoskeletal pain with widespread hypersensitivity to bright light, touch, noise, pesticides, mechanical pressure, medications, and high and low temperatures. Abnormalities in metabolic, biochemical, hormonal, immune-regulatory, and CNS are likely to be affected with central sensitization. The characteristics of central sensitivity include pain disproportionate to the injury or sensory amplification and sensory and motor cortical representation changes, which result in perceptual changes in body images. Often, even thinking about movement can cause pain, symptoms can spread outside of the injured area, and there are abnormal movement patterns and abnormal sensations along with maladaptive psychosocial traits. Nijs and colleagues[16] describe that pressure pain thresholds at sites not anatomically related elicit widespread symptoms, distribution, and persistent central sensitization. In an article by Smart and coworkers[17] looking at a discriminative validity study, three symptoms and one sign emerged as a predictive classification of central back pain (sensitivity 91.8 and specificity 97.7) These symptoms and signs were (1) disproportionate, nonmechanical unpredictable patterns of pain provocation in response to multiple/nonspecific aggravating/easing factors; (2) pain disproportionate to the nature and extent of injury or pathology; (3) maladaptive psychosocial factors (eg, negative emotions, poor self-efficacy, maladaptive beliefs and pain behaviors); and (4) altered family/work/social life and medical conflict.

Central sensitization manifests as pain hypersensitivity, particularly tactile allodynia, pressure hyperalgesia, and after sensations. In central sensitization stimuli that should not be painful can now activate nociceptors and are painful. This is the pain from the "wind blowing on the arm." Many researchers have identified that the pain is from central changes, distorting or amplifying the pain. One way of simplifying central sensitization for a patient is to describe this as a problem with volume control, even small quiet signals are now being processed as painfully loud.

There are several physical examination findings that can be attributed to central sensitization and help the clinician with diagnosis. There are changes in sensory perceptions and disturbances in limb perception. For example, two-point discrimination and vibratory changes occur. The changes are caused by reorganization of the body schema in the brain.[18,19] Patients can also have bilateral widespread decrease with pressure pain threshold. These bilateral changes have been clearly shown in patients with unilateral carpal tunnel. These side-to-side changes suggest a dysfunction in a central processing mechanism.[18] Often patients with central sensitization fail to respond to peripheral interventions because the central mechanism has not been addressed. Thus for these patients recognition and treatment of the central components is critical. Other than the clinical signs and symptoms of central sensitization there is not a definitive test by which it can be identified.

TREATMENT OF PAIN MECHANISMS

Pizzo and Clark[20] presented a roadmap for relieving pain in America. First they recommend recognition that pain results from biologic, psychological, and social factors. Next, treatment requires a comprehensive approach to prevention and management. Finally, change must begin with the education of the person in pain and recognition that beliefs about pain can substantially affect outcomes. The effectiveness of pain treatments depends greatly on the strength of the clinician-patient relationship (**Box 1**).

Effective treatment of pain requires a holistic strategy addressing the multifactorial mechanisms causing pain. It is well known that stress plays a significant role in the exacerbation of pain and other physical symptoms. The patient with pain must have the tools to regulate the stress and this involves good emotional thoughts and healthy behaviors to limit catastrophic thinking and dwelling on the pain.[21] The patient must understand and be in control so cognitive modulation of pain through positive expectation, belief, attention, and limiting catastrophic thinking can be effective. Priganc and Stralka[22] found that successful treatment of patients in pain requires a bottom-up peripheral treatment plan and a central top-down

---

Box 1
A blueprint for transforming pain

Pain results from biologic, psychological, and social factors.

Treatment requires comprehensive integrated approaches to management.

Change must begin with the education of a person in pain and recognition that beliefs of pain can substantially affect outcomes.

Adapted from Pizzo PA, Clark NM. Alleviating suffering 101: pain relief in the United States. N Engl J Med 2012;366(3):197–9.

plan. Bottom-up treatment is treating the peripheral symptoms, such as edema, stiffness, and lack of range of motion. Top-down treatment consists of identifying any changes in the CNS and using mirror therapy or graded motor imagery in treatment. Research over the last 20 years strongly suggests that this holistic approach is a component of proper care and good outcomes.

Treatment of Peripheral Nociceptive and Inflammatory Mechanism

Interventions for management of all pain start with thoroughly educating the patient on the underlying reasons behind the inflammatory and pain symptoms. Woolf[4] describes the pain neural process classification as if pain were a fire alarm. Nociceptive pain is activated by a hot fire, inflammatory pain is activated by warm temperatures, and pathologic (prolonged persistent) pain is a false alarm. Giving the patient this framework allows the patient to better understand the different components to their pain.

Before treatment an upper quadrant evaluation is performed. This provides information on the tissue status that can direct what modalities are appropriate. Modalities or physical agents can be used to increase blood flow in hopes of increasing healing, to control edema, and to modulate pain. Before the use of modalities, the upper quadrant evaluation assists in choosing the correct intervention for safe use on the upper extremity.

The treatment of peripheral pain generators often uses a bottom-up strategy. Bottom-up treatment addresses the peripheral symptoms of pain, swelling, inflammation, limited motion, joint protection, and muscle weakness. Common techniques to treat peripheral/inflammatory pain are thermal agents, electrotherapy techniques, and physical modalities. Physical modalities control edema, facilitate tissue healing, and modulate pain. The program should progress to include joint protection as needed; rest; and activity modification using the active exercise-oriented approach of improving motion, developing normal movement patterns, and emphasizing activities to assist in functional outcomes. For the most effect, the patient must be actively involved in treatment and compliant with home exercises for relaxation and mindfulness. Soft tissue mobilization along with manual therapy has been supported by empirical evidence to be helpful in the treatment of nociceptive pain. Beyond physical manipulation of the tissues, treatment of nociceptive mechanisms may also include different modalities, such as heat, cold, therapeutic ultrasound, transcutaneous electrical nerve stimulation, interferential

current, and laser therapy. Physical agents should never be used alone and should be considered as part of a comprehensive hand rehabilitation program. Unfortunately, in some patients the pain is not proportional to the amount of tissue damage and likely involves significant psychosocial variables and CNS changes. These patients with severe pain acutely are at more risk of a slow or poor recovery. The treatment of nociceptive mechanisms and prognosis should follow a predictable pattern of recovery as tissue heals and inflammation diminishes.

Treatment of Peripheral Neurogenic Symptoms

Treatment of pain generated through peripheral neurogenic symptoms also needs to be multifaceted. First, nerves need adequate blood supply, space to move, and a healthy soft tissue bed to stay healthy or to recover after injury. Peripheral nervous system structures must be able to freely move to accommodate different limb positions. Following injury to a nerve the usual healing process may make movement of that nerve painful. Thus, treatment begins with upper limb neurodynamic testing to locate sources of nerve tension and to identify what structures are involved. Upper limb neurodynamic testing places the upper limb through a series of movements to place mechanical forces on the nerves. Specific tests that cause pain help the practioner identify sources of pain.[23] The level of nerve irritability must be identified before movement of the entire upper extremity is initiated.

My strategies for peripheral neurogenic pain are aimed at elongating the nerve and decreasing pressure around the nerve. It is not usual to find posture imbalances and tight musculature causing nerve symptoms and the upper limb neurodynamics test assists in locating these. Once the sites of entrapment are identified, then nerve gliding is determined according to the irritability of that nerve. Finally, for the treatment of patients with alteration in perception, the therapy should include graded motor imagery and mirror therapy.

Treatment of Central Sensitization Mechanism

Treatment of central pain mechanisms needs to account for the multiple areas contributing to the pain. According to functional MRI, multiple areas within the CNS show cortical organization changes and altered activity from the dorsal horn of the spinal cord to many brain regions. Treatment of central sensitization needs to move beyond common modalities. Treating central sensitization needs to focus on the brain changes following cortical representation. Treatment must be targeted toward eliminating musculoskeletal dysfunction and aberrant central pain processing, along with therapy addressing the physiologic and psychological processing of pain. To address the neuroplastic changes in sensory-motor areas, activities should be stimulus driven, performed for short periods of time, and repetitive. McManus[21] and associates developed active self-management strategies for the CNS changes, which consist of mindful awareness, cognitive behavioral therapy, graded motor imagery, exercise, pleasant activity scheduling, and sleep management.

The patient should be continually reminded that pain with movement does not mean tissue damage, it is just the brain's abnormal processing, and that being sore is a part of rehabilitation. Graded motor imagery techniques as developed by Moseley and coworkers[24] use sequential brain-training techniques of left/right identification, motor imagery exercises, and mirror therapy in rehabilitation of persistent pain and central sensitization. Many hand and upper extremity patients have pain, difficulty in moving and initiating movement, or fear of moving, and graded motor imagery may be beneficial for these patients. Bowering and coworkers[25] report that novel approaches, such as mirror therapy and graded motor imagery, to address these neuroplastic changes show promise.

There is some evidence to suggest that patient education about the neurobiology of pain might improve illness beliefs and movement performance and lessen the threat value of pain. Louw and coworkers[26] report that education on persistent musculoskeletal pain may positively impact pain, disability, catastrophizing, and physical performance. Patient neuroscience education might also lessen the cognitive-affective contributions by reducing facilitation or enhancing inhibition of descending pain pathways. The neuroscience educational component must be easily understood by the patient and reinforced by the therapist working on their hand injury to receive optimal outcomes.

Often treatment of these complex patients requires multiple disciplines within the health care field. Treating central pain requires nonpharmacologic and pharmacologic management. Often patients have been misdiagnosed or undiagnosed and the longevity of their symptoms has caused frustration, depression, and anxiety. With the team approach all aspects of treatment must be considered, such as identifying the need for antidepressants or antianxiety drugs along with nerve membrane stabilization. Psychological interventions, such as cognitive behavior training, must be considered and may be necessary before therapy is initiated.

Box 2
"Yellow flags" reflecting maladaptive psychological response to pain/injury

Beliefs, appraisals, judgment

Unhealthy beliefs that injury is uncontrollable or likely to worsen

Expectation of poor treatment outcomes

Delayed return to work

Emotional responses

Excessive worries, fears, and anxiety but not meeting criteria for diagnosis of mental disorder

Pain behavior (including coping strategies)

Avoidance of activities because of expectations

Overreliance on passive treatments (hot packs, cold packs, analgesic)

Adapted from Nicholas MK, Linton SJ. Early identification and management of psychological risk factors (yellow flags) in patients with low back pain: a reappraisal. Phys Ther 2011;91(5):737–53.

There must be an open relationship with everyone on the interdisciplinary team and with the patient to avoid increasing symptoms and frustration of everyone. Clinicians must select treatment of central sensitization to target the neurophysiologic mechanisms and improve outcomes. Nicholas and Linton[27] provide examples of some "yellow flags" that may suggest the presence of undetermined psychosocial risk factors that impact care (**Box 2**). Providers should try to identify these psychosocial factors early so that all appropriate interventions are offered to help treat the pain.

For all the interventions listed in this article, there is limited scientific evidence. There is a clear need for more information on how clinicians treat pain. Future research is needed to continue advancement of the field.

SUMMARY

Pain is a multidimensional experience generated by the complex interactions of the "body-self neuromatrix."[28] Thus, clinical treatment must be directed at the sensory inputs and other components from other nerve entrapments to central components, such as stress, as maladaptive behaviors. Recent findings suggest that in rehabilitation of persistent pain the neuroplastic changes in the CNS must be addressed for a good functional outcome. Patients must be educated and empowered and an active participant in their treatment. Cognitive-based education interventions that involve the patient understanding the pain processing and mechanisms, changing their faulty beliefs regarding pain, and understanding the importance of movement yield better outcomes.

REFERENCES

1. Elliott M, Barbe M. Understanding pain mechanisms: the basis of clinical decision making for pain modulation. In: Skirven T, Osterman AL, Fedorczyk JM, et al, editors. Rehabilitation of the Hand and Upper Extremity, vol. 6. [chapter 113]. Philadelphia: Elsevier (Mosby); 2011. p. 1449–69.

2. Fedorczyk JM. Pain management: principles of therapist intervention. In: Skirven T, Osterman AL, Fedorczyk JM, et al, editors. Rehabilitation of the Hand and Upper Extremity, vol. 6. [chapter 114]. Philadelphia: Elsevier (Mosby); 2011. p. 1461–9.

3. Butler DS. The sensitive nervous system: pain mechanisms and peripheral sensitivity [Chapter 3]. Adelaide (Australia): NOI Group Publication; 2012. p. 47–72.

4. Woolf CJ. Central sensitization: implication for the diagnosis and treatment of pain. Pain 2011; 152(suppl):S2–15.

5. Pain and gate control. In: Wall P, Melzack R, editors. Textbook of pain. 4th edition. Philadelphia: Saunders.

6. Sluka KA. Definitions, concepts and models of pain [Chapter 1]. In: Sluka KA, editor. Mechanisms and management of pain for the physical therapist. IASP Pres; 2009. p. 3–18.

7. Shacklock M. Clinical neurodynamics. A new system of musculoskeletal treatment [Chapter 4]. Canada: Elsevier; 2005. p. 1–30.

8. Upton A, McComas AJ. The double crush syndrome in nerve entrapment. Lancet 1973;1:359–61.

9. Latremoliere A, Woolf C. Central sensitization: a generator of pain hypersensitivity by central neural plasticity. J Pain 2009;10(9):895–926.

10. Quintero L, Cardenas R, Suarez-Roca H. Stress induced hyperalgesia is associated with a reduced and delayed GABA inhibitory control that enhances post-synaptic NDMA receptor activation in the spinal cord. Pain 2011;152(8):1909–22.

11. Pelteeier R, Higgins J, Bourbonnais D. Is neuroplasticity in the central nervous system the missing link to our understanding of chronic musculoskeletal disorders? BMC Musculoskelet Disord 2015;16:25.

12. Rosen B, Vikstrom P, Turner S, et al. Enhanced early sensory outcome after nerve repair as a result of immediate post-operative relearning: a randomized controlled trial. J Hand Surg Eur Vol 2015;40(6): 598–606.

13. May A. Chronic pain may change the structure of the brain. Pain 2008;137(1):7–15.

14. Toas H, Galea MP, Hodges PW, et al. Reorganization of the motor cortex is associated with postural control deficits in recurrent low back pain. Brain 2008; 131(Pt 8):2161–71.

15. Mailinen S, Hlushchuk Y, Koskinen M, et al. Aberrant temporal and spatial activity during rest in patients with chronic pain. Proc Natl Acad Sci U S A 2010; 107(14):6493–7.

16. Nijs J, van Wilgen CP, Van Oosterwijck J, et al. How to explain central sensitization to patients with "unexplained"chronic pain. Pharmacotherapy 2011; 12(7):1087–98.

17. Smart KM, Blake C, Staines A, et al. The discriminative validity of nociceptive, peripheral neuropathic, and central sensitization as mechanisms-based classifications of musculoskeletal pain. Clin J Pain 2011;27(8):655–63.

18. Schmidt S, Current concepts in pain management: merging manual therapy and pain science. Scientific Presentation: Combined APTA Section Meeting. San Diego, CA, January, 2012.

19. Fernandez C, De-la Llave Rincon A, Cuadrado M, et al. Bilateral widespread mechanical pain sensitivity in carpal tunnel syndrome: evidence of central processing in unilateral neuropathy. Brain 2009;132:1472–9.

20. Pizzo PA, Clark NM. Alleviating suffering 101-pain relief in the United States. N Engl J Med 2012; 366(3):197–9.

21. McManus C, The pain puzzle: empowering the patient to put the pieces together. Presented at the American Physical Therapy Conference. Charlotte (NC), June 12, 2014.

22. Priganc VW, Stralka SW. Graded motor imagery. J Hand Ther 2011;24(2):164–8.

23. Nee RJ, Jull GA, Vicenzino B, et al. The validity of upper-limb neurodynamic tests for detecting peripheral neuropathic pain. J Orthop Sports Phys Ther 2012;42(5):413–24.

24. Moseley LG, Butler DS, Beames TB, et al. The graded motor imagery book. Adelaide (Australia): NOI Publications; 2012.

25. Bowering KJ, O'Connell NE, Tabor A, et al. The effects of graded motor imagery and its components on chronic pain: a systematic review and meta-analysis. J Pain 2013;14(1):3–13.

26. Louw A, Diener I, Butler D, et al. The effect of neuroscience education on pain, disability, anxiety and stress in chronic musculoskeletal pain. Arch Phys Med Rehabil 2011;92(12):2041–56.

27. Nicholas MK, Linton SJ. Early identification and management of psychological risk factors (yellow flags) in patients with low back pain: a reappraisal. Phys Ther 2011;91(5):737–53.

28. Melzack R. Evolution of the neuromatrix theory of pain: first presented at the third world congress of World Institute of Pain. May 2005. Pain Pract 2005; 5(2):85–9.

Surgical Treatment of Upper Extremity Pain

Arnold Lee Dellon, MD, PhD

KEYWORDS

- Neuroma • Nerve compression • Complex regional pain syndrome • Reflex sympathetic dystrophy
- Joint pain

KEY POINTS

Critical steps in surgical treatment of hand/upper extremity pain

1. History suggests injury to nerve.
2. Physical examination consistent with nerve injury.
   a. Positive Tinel sign at site of nerve injury or compression.
   b. Pain with joint movement.
   c. Altered sensation.
3. Nerve block.
   a. Results in loss of sensation in the skin territory of interest.
   b. Relieves pain, and if not, then a second nerve must be blocked.
4. Permits pain-free joint movement, increased grip strength.
5. Surgical treatment.
   a. Neuromas are resected.
   b. Nerve compressions are released.
   c. Proximal end of divided nerves is implanted into muscle.
   d. Partial joint denervation is done.

INTRODUCTION

The current approach to surgical treatment of the painful hand and upper extremity stems from basic science and translational research from the early 1980s. This research focused on why dorsoradial wrist pain had such a high rate of treatment failure. Typically these patients would have a dorsal wrist ganglion excision or release of the first dorsal extensor compartment to treat extensor tenosynovitis and have postoperative pain over the dorsoradial aspect of the wrist/hand, the territory of the radial sensory nerve. The classic teaching for this problem was: do not disturb the "mature end-bulb neuroma," but move it to a different location. The problem was that these patients had a radial sensory nerve neuroma but a treatment plan of moving the neuroma to a new location without resecting the neuroma would *not* relieve the pain. There were several reasons for treatment failures including (1) the in-continuity or mature end-bulb neuroma was the source of the pain signals and had to be resected,[1] (2) the initial surgical site represented an overlap of the radial sensory nerve and the lateral antebrachial cutaneous nerve in 75% of people,[2] and (3) resecting a nerve and leaving the proximal end in the subcutaneous tissue near a joint resulted in recurrent neuroma formation.

Thus a different strategy was required. Research suggested that implanting the resected nerve end into muscle optimized the environment where the nerve attempts regeneration.[3,4] Using

Department of Plastic Surgery, Johns Hopkins University, 1122 Kenilworth Drive, Suite 18, Towson, MD 21204, USA
E-mail address: ALDellon@Dellon.com

Hand Clin 32 (2016) 71–80
http://dx.doi.org/10.1016/j.hcl.2015.08.008

this new research, an algorithm was created for treatment of the painful hand that has withstood the test of time (**Fig. 1**).[5–11] This algorithm is outlined in the Key Points. The same algorithm also applies to lower extremity pain.[12–15]

PATIENT PRESENTATION

Patients with nerve pain typically present in four ways, outlined next.

Typical Presentation One: The Cutaneous Neuroma

In this scenario surgical intervention has resulted in a painful scar. There are several common examples of cutaneous neuromas in the upper limb surgeon's practice. **Table 1** highlights common nerves injured during upper limb exposures. These patients typically come to the office and the surgeons' challenge is to recognize that the pain is from a cutaneous neuroma, and not from recurrence of the pathology that necessitated the initial procedure.

Typical Presentation Two: Nerve Compression

Although hand surgeons are expert at recognizing chronic peripheral nerve compression, they may overlook this diagnosis in the setting of diffuse pain with a history of multiple interventions or a patient with a diagnosis of complex regional pain syndrome (CRPS). Another diagnostic problem is that acute nerve compression typically causes more pain compared with chronic nerve compression.[17,18] Neurolysis of compressed peripheral nerves can relieve pain and even successfully treat the patient with CRPS.[19]

Typical Presentation Three: Joint Pain

The classic teaching is that joint pain is related to a biomechanical problem with bone, ligament, and/or cartilage of the painful joint. Clearly this is true and almost always the source of the pain. It

is also true classically that anatomy books do not have illustrations of the innervations of any upper extremity joint or lower extremity joint. If joints are not innervated, how can any joint be a source of pain? Although total wrist denervated was reported in the second issue of *Journal of Hand Surgery* in 1977,[20] the approach was more a destructive cauterization of ligaments than a true identification and removal of individual nerves. The failures in this total wrist denervation approach were in those patients with unstable wrists, who went on to require partial wrist arthrodesis, confirming that biomechanical factors must be corrected before any attempt to relieve joint pain of neural origin. In 1979, the approach to identifying the posterior interosseous nerve was described,[21] and in 1984 the approach to identifying the anterior interosseous nerve was described.[22] The typical situation is that a person has fallen on to an outstretched wrist, and has persistent pain despite appropriate treatment of the skeletal abnormalities. If wrist movement still hurts or is limited by pain, the diagnosis must include joint pain of neural origin. For the wrist joint, this includes the differential diagnosis of injury to the terminal branch of the posterior interosseous nerve or the anterior interosseous nerve, which is determined with differential diagnostic nerve blocks. Then, based on which of these gives pain relief, or perhaps both nerves had to be blocked, the surgical approach to treat this wrist pain is to resect the distal posterior interosseous nerve,[23] the anterior interosseous nerve,[22] or both (see **Fig. 3**).[24] Reviews of the operative approach to the joint afferents to the upper[25] and lower extremity joints[26,27] and the outcomes of nerve resections have been published. Techniques to joint denervation are discussed later.[28–32] There has been concern that denervation would adversely impact the joints. Studies on the joint afferents and their effect on reflexes and proprioception have concluded that partial joint denervation does not cause dysfunction.[33–36]

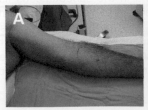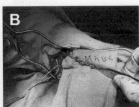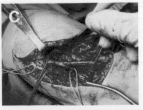

Fig. 1. (*A*) Patient with chronic pain syndrome after vascular surgery in antebrachial region, trigger points noted by the asterisks and the *incisions* from the intervention marked. (*B*) The neuroma of the medial antebrachial nerve is on the background material. After resection of the neuroma, the proximal end was implanted into the medial head of the triceps muscle. (*C*) Neurolysis of the swollen median nerve (*red vessel loops*) included the anterior interosseous nerve (*distal blue loop*). The ulnar nerve is noted within the proximal blue vessel loop.

Table 1
Common nerves injured during upper limb exposures

Incision Site	Inciting Procedures	Potential Injured Nerve
Dorsoradial wrist[3,9]	Release of extensor tenosynovitis Dorsal wrist ganglion excision	Radial sensory nerve Lateral antebrachial cutaneous nerve or both
Palmar[11]	Open carpal tunnel release Endoscopic carpal tunnel release	Palmar cutaneous branch of the median nerve
Medial elbow[6]	Cubital tunnel	Medial antebrachial cutaneous nerve (see **Fig. 1**) Medial brachial cutaneous nerve
Lateral epicondyle[16]	Tennis elbow repair	Posterior cutaneous nerve of the forearm

Data from Refs.[3,6,9,11,16]

Typical Presentation Four: Complex Regional Pain Syndrome

The patient with CRPS presents after an injury or an elective surgery. Their clinical picture is of chronic pain that exceeds the distribution of a single peripheral nerve, vascular changes, hand swelling, and disuse. These patients need long-term pain management and often have concomitant anxiety/depression, drug addiction, and disability. In this article, the position is taken that CRPS is from a combination of nerve injuries: underlying neuroma, nerve compression, or joint afferent injury. The surgical approach to these injured nerves described in this article can help these challenging patients achieve long-term pain relief and improved extremity function.[19,37] CRPS can be improved by surgical intervention addressing the nerve injury that is generating the pain.

DIAGNOSTIC TESTING: NERVE BLOCKS

The best way to determine if a particular nerve is the source of the patient's perceived pain is to stop that nerve from functioning temporarily by doing a diagnostic nerve block. The hand surgeon can often do these in the office, although there are times when colleagues, such as a pain management doctor, may be asked to perform the nerve block. This includes (1) when a patient requires the block to be at the nerve root level, (2) when the patient or the insurance company or the surgeon wishes someone independent from the treating hand surgeon to do the nerve block, (3) complex anatomy in which ultrasound localization might be helpful, or (4) if the patient requires intravenous sedation and needs to be done in an operating room setting with an anesthesiologist present (the hand surgeon can perform blocks in the operating room if it is so desired).

The following list the technical steps to performing successful blocks:

1. Be sure the patient is not allergic to the local anesthetic agent (these are usually amides, and if the patient is allergic to these there is still the possibility to do the block with procaine, which is not an amide).
2. Ensure the injection site localizes only one nerve (recall that the radial sensory and the lateral antebrachial cutaneous nerves overlap in the region of the anatomic snuff box).
3. Inject adjacent to the nerve, not in the nerve, and state this in the report.
4. Record the preblock pain level, grip and pinch strength, and joint range of motion and record these again postblock.
5. Ensure that the desired skin territory had decreased sensation after the block.
6. Request the patient to report back on the results of the block the following day. Having the patient create an hourly pain diary is a good idea.
7. Be prepared to do a second and third block either the same office visit or at a subsequent one until all the nerves contributing to the pain are identified.
8. Be prepared for vasovagal episodes.
9. Monitor the patient 15 minutes after the block.

NERVE COMPRESSION

Hand surgeons are uniquely trained to do nerve decompressions in the upper extremity, and it is beyond the scope of this article to discus how to decompress upper extremity nerves. From the point of view of hand pain, it must be emphasized again that chronic compression is part of the spectrum of diagnoses presenting as hand pain and that surgical intervention is an appropriate treatment modality. The hand surgeon should be certain to look and examine for some of the more rare forms of nerve compression, such as radial sensory nerve compression in the forearm,[38] pronator syndrome, and brachial plexus compression in the thoracic inlet.[39,40]

NEUROMA PAIN: NERVE RECONSTRUCTION

Hand pain caused by an injury to a critically important nerve should be treated by resection of the neuroma-in-continuity and reconstruction of the nerve. An example is pain in the wrist and numbness in several fingers after a median nerve injury (**Fig. 2**). After surgery, there can be pain related to neural regeneration, which is often different than the preoperative pain. This is treated with neuropathic pain medication, such as gabapentin, and with techniques of sensory re-education.[41,42] It is important to make the patient aware that these sensations are normal and have a discrete duration.

NEUROMA PAIN: NEUROMA RESECTION AND MUSCLE IMPLANTATION

If the pain generator is an expendable nerve, neuroma resection can be considered. First the pain must be relieved by diagnostic nerve block and the patient must understand and accept the trade of permanent numbness for pain relief. Once the offending nerve has been identified, a plan must be developed depending on the anatomic location. The goals are to place the neuroma in a position under no tension, not crossing a joint line, and with adequate soft tissue coverage. A neuroma located at or proximal to the wrist must be resected and the proximal end implanted into a muscle with minimal excursion. This limits stretching on the implanted nerve during movement of that

muscle. The brachioradialis is a good example of such a muscle and is an excellent location to implant the radial sensory nerve, the lateral antebrachial cutaneous nerve, or both of them.[9] However, if the lateral antebrachial cutaneous nerve is injured just distal to the elbow, then the nerve must be implanted proximal to the joint, into the brachialis muscle (**Fig. 3**).

The palmar cutaneous branch of the median nerve can easily be buried into the pronator quadratus.[11] The medial antebrachial cutaneous nerve and the medial brachial cutaneous nerves go easily into the medial head of the triceps (**Fig. 4**).[43]

The posterior cutaneous nerve of the forearm goes easily into the lateral head of the triceps.[16] The dorsal cutaneous branch of the ulnar nerve goes easily into the flexor carpi ulnaris. Placement of the nerve end is performed with care. The proximal end must be sufficiently long to implant about 1.0 to 1.5 cm of it into the muscle. A small "Crile" type clamp is pushed gently into the muscle to create a tunnel that angles proximally. Then that clamp is used to loosely grasp the end of the nerve and implant it into the tunnel. A suture is not used to secure the "nerve" so that a new injury to the nerve is not created.

A digital nerve neuroma represents a problem with this strategy, because there are no sufficiently bulky muscles in the hand into which to implant a nerve. The primary treatment of a digital neuroma should be to reconstruct that nerve. However, in the situation where there is a distal amputation, the proximal end of the nerve must be placed somewhere. Implantation into the medullary cavity of the metacarpal is one choice. A microsurgical approach can be considered, which could be an end-to-side reconstruction into an adjacent common volar digital nerve, which could be thought

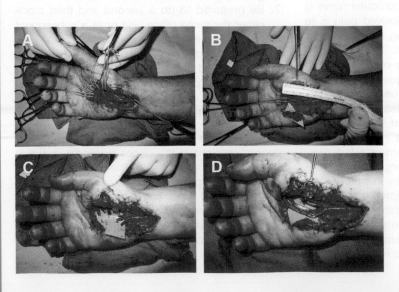

Fig. 2. Patient was 18 months following an endoscopic carpal tunnel release and had lost sensation in the thumb and index finger, and lost motor function. (*A*) At surgery, the digital nerve branches of the median nerve are encircled in *vessel loops*, as is the proximal median nerve. (*B*) The neuroma-in-continuity is resected, permitting salvage of the intact common volar digital nerves to the index/middle webspace and to the middle/ring webspace. (*C*) Each of the nerve ends to be connected is seen resting on the *blue background material*. (*D*) Nerve allograft was used as the interposition nerve graft.

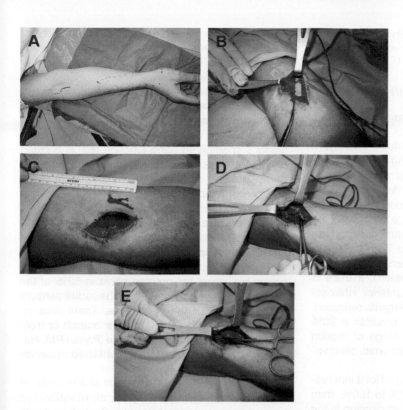

Fig. 3. Patient with hand pain related to a stretch/traction injury of the lateral antebrachial cutaneous (LABC) nerve at the region of the elbow. (*A*) The location of the pain is outlined, and block of the LABC in the forearm confirmed the LABC as pain generator. Radial sensory nerve block gave no relief. (*B*) The LABC can have a proximal branch, as shown here, and each must be resected as shown in (*C*). The proximal end of the LABC must have a neurolysis to above the antecubital fossa (*D*) and then it can be turned and implanted into the brachialis muscle proximal to the elbow (*E*).

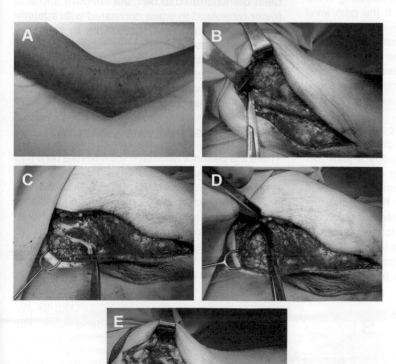

Fig. 4. (*A*) Ulnar nerve transposition places the medial antebrachial cutaneous (MABC) nerve and the medial brachial cutaneous (MAB) at risk for injury. (*B*) the MABC must be identified, the neuroma resected, and (*C*) the proximal end implanted into the medial head of the triceps muscle. (*D*) The same approach, after the neurolysis of the ulnar nerve is completed, is used for the neuroma of the MAB, and it too is implanted into the medial head of the triceps muscle (*E*).

of as an implantation of the nerve into another nerve. This has been reported experimentally[44] and clinically.[45]

JOINT PAIN OF NEURAL ORIGIN

A common joint pain problem is wrist pain following a sprain or distal radius fracture. Once it is clear that there is ligamentous stability, a healed fracture, and any irritating hardware has been removed, then the residual pain with wrist dorsiflexion or flexion is most likely caused by injury to the posterior or anterior interosseous nerves. To confirm this diagnosis, a set of preblock wrist range of motion is obtained and grip strength with the elbow in 90° of flexion. Then the nerve block is done to the posterior interosseous nerve, and the measurements are repeated. If there is some remaining pain, then the anterior interosseous is blocked and the measurements repeated. A good response to the block predicts a 90% improvement in wrist pain and range of motion after the partial dorsal and/or volar wrist denervation (**Fig. 5**).

If the nerve block of the suspected joint innervation relieves the patient's pain 90% to 100%, then there should be no other nerve participating in the pain perception from that joint. If the pain level drops after the block from, for example, an eight to a five, then there is still another nerve participating. For the wrist joint, after the posterior interosseous nerve and anterior interosseous nerve have been blocked, pain remaining is either radial or ulnar, and innervation of that side of the wrist joint must then be blocked.

Radial- or ulnar-sided wrist pain presents a more challenging problem. The differential diagnosis for these hardly ever incudes a joint afferent. Consider ulnar-sided wrist pain related to a torn triangular fibrocartilage complex. There is a hole in the cartilage and the therapeutic approach is to repair the hole, instead of considering that the pain is related to nerve injured during the process of tearing the triangular fibrocartilage complex. The innervation of the triangular fibrocartilage complex has been described

recently and involves several different nerves, requiring careful differential nerve blocks.[31] Each of these involved nerves can be resected if necessary (**Fig. 6**).

Similarly, radial-sided wrist pain, especially of the first carpometacarpal joint, can be approached in the same manner. Instead of a resection/implant arthroplasty, or a fusion, which may limit a professional's specialized hand function (eg, in a piano player), it is possible to remove a painful volar bone spur and denervate the volar capsule of the first carpometacarpal joint (**Fig. 7**).

In an unpublished study, using 3.5-loupe magnification on nine fresh cadaver wrists, the radial-sided dissection identified innervation by the lateral antebrachial cutaneous nerve in 100% of the specimens, innervation by the palmar cutaneous branch of the median nerve in 82% of the specimens, and innervation by the radial sensory nerve in 18% of the specimens. There was no innervation from the thenar motor branch or from the deep branch of the ulnar nerve (Parikh PM, Hashemi S, Murphy MS, et al, unpublished observations, 2010).

Proceeding to a more proximal site of pain, at the lateral humeral epicondyle a denervation has been demonstrated to be more effective and with faster rehabilitation when compared with a lateral epicondylectomy, allowing patients to return to activity, such as tennis.[3,29] Most recently, a similar approach has been shown to be effective in one baseball pitcher with medial humeral epicondylitis.[28,33] Dennervation procedures are another surgical tool to treat painful joints.

COMPLEX REGIONAL PAIN SYNDROME

There are patients who have such severe pain that it dominates their life and that of their loved ones. When this was described by Silas Weir Mitchell, a neurologist studying nerve injuries during and after the US Civil War, the pain was caused predominantly by the round musket ball causing a partial division of a single peripheral nerve.[46] Mitchell coined the term "causalgia" to describe this demoralizing burning pain, requiring the soldier to

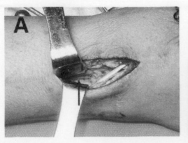 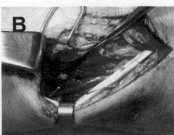

Fig. 5. Intraoperative view of partial dorsal wrist denervation with the posterior interosseous nerve (*arrow*) (*A*) and partial volar wrist denervation through the same incision with the anterior interosseous nerve demonstrated by the Freer elevator (*B*).

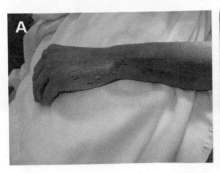
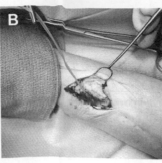

Fig. 6. Patient who had ulnar wrist pain after injury to the triangular fibrocartilage complex and multiple surgeries to relieve pain. (A) She ultimately had creation of a "one bone forearm" yet remained disabled because of ulnar sided wrist pain with any attempt to flex the wrist and whenever the dorsal ulnar side of the hand was touched. (B) Intraoperative view demonstrates the innervation of the triangular fibrocartilage complex area as a branch of the dorsal ulnar cutaneous nerve. Both of these were resected and the proximal end implanted into the flexor carpi ulnaris muscle. This procedure relieved the debilitating ulnar-sided wrist pain.

protect the affected part even from the breeze. When the pain is outside or greater than the distribution of a single nerve, the term "reflex sympathetic dystrophy" (RSD) comes into use. Often this occurs after a trivial injury, such as a sprained wrist, or a simple surgery, such as a carpal tunnel release or open fixation of a distal radius fracture. I like to say that RSD is an acronym for "Really Stupid Diagnosis."[47] This is because the diffuse pain can be caused by a combination of one or more individual nerve injuries, such as an injured joint afferent from the sprain, a compressed median nerve from the swelling and immobilization, and perhaps also a damaged radial sensory nerve from the external fixation device.

Until recently there has been no scientific support in terms of an outcome study of the surgical approach to the treatment of CRPS. In 2010, a prospective study was published where 100 consecutive patients with the diagnosis of RSD or CRPS were accrued and evaluated for the presence of multiple peripheral nerve pain triggers.[37] The examination included a Tinel evaluation of

involved nerves, and nerve blocks of involved nerves (Fig. 8).

Of the 100 patients, there were 70 that responded to the blocks and had a surgical approach to the treatment of their pain. Forty of these were upper and 30 were lower extremity nerve patients. Table 2 presents the painful nerves treated in this study. The outcomes for this study were decreased pain medication usage and improvement in recovery of function. For the upper extremity patients, at a mean of 28 months follow-up, the results were excellent in 40%, good in 40%, and failure in 20%. In the lower extremity, at a mean of 23 months follow-up, the results were excellent in 47%, good in 33%, and failure 20% (Fig. 9). It was concluded that most patients referred with a diagnosis of CRPS I (RSD) have continuing pain input from injured joint or cutaneous afferents and/or nerve compressions, and therefore similar to a patient with CRPS II (causalgia) they can be treated successfully with an appropriate peripheral nerve surgical strategy.[37]

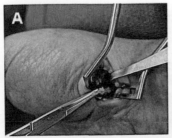
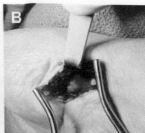
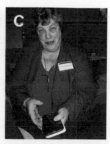

Fig. 7. Denervation of the carpometacarpal joint for radial-volar first metacarpal-carpal pain. The patient had typical radiograph findings for first carpometacarpal joint osteoarthritis, but the pain was radial volar rather than dorsoradial. (A) Intraoperative view of nerve innervating this aspect of the joint that was resected. (B) Intraoperative view showing joint space after resecting the volar bone spur. (C) Ten-year follow-up of the patient using thumbs to use a smartphone.

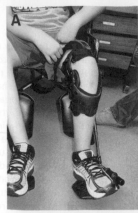
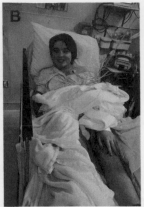
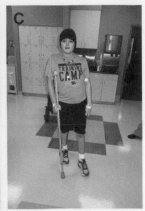

Fig. 8. Because hand surgeons are comfortable identifying and treating peripheral nerve injuries they are also called to treat nerves in the lower limb. A 13 year old is 18 months after a snowboarding accident caused disabling left knee pain. The skin of the knee and below the knee cannot be touched without severe pain and he cannot bend his knee without severe pain. (*A*) He uses a knee brace, crutches, and a wheel chair. Nerve blocks were done using intravenous sedation of the lateral retinacular nerve and the proximal tibiofibular joint, and the medial cutaneous nerve of the thigh, the infrapatellar branch of the saphenous nerve, and the medial retinacular nerve. Following these blocks, he could (*B*) touch the skin without pain, bend the knee, and (*C*) ambulate on one crutch, demonstrating that the CRPS was caused by multiple peripheral nerve pain inputs.

Table 2
Nerves treated in patients with CRPS

	Upper Limb (n)	Lower Limb (n)
Neurolysis	Brachial plexus (2)	Common peroneal (10), superficial peroneal (5)
	Carpal tunnel (5)	Deep peroneal (1)
	Cubital tunnel (9)	Interdigital nerve (1)
	Radial sensory (9)	Medial ankle tunnels for the tibial nerve (10)
Joints denervated	Elbow (1)	Knee (3)
	Wrist (4)	Ankle (1)
Neuromas resected	Radial sensory (5)	Superficial peroneal nerve (2)
	Lateral antebrachial (7)	Saphenous (8)
	Posterior cutaneous nerve of the forearm (3)	Sural (2)
		Medial calcaneal nerves (3)
	Medial brachial (1)	
	Medial antebrachial nerves (2)	
Neuromas repaired	Digital nerve (1)	—

From Dellon AL, Andronian E, Rosson GD. Lower extremity CRPS: long-term results of surgical treatment of peripheral nerve pain generators. J Foot Ankle Surg 2010;49:35; with permission.

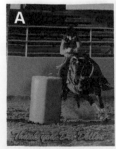
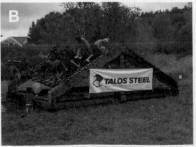
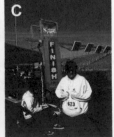

Fig. 9. Surgically treated patients with CRPS can have durable results. (*A*) Two years after a rodeo riding crush injury to her left leg, a patient has returned to barrel racing and won her division. (*B*) Three years after ankle injury, a patient has returned to full activity, here (in the pink scarf at the top) competing in a Mudder Race. (*C*) Five years after ankle injury, a patient is completing a 5K race.

SUMMARY

Surgery as a treatment of neuropathic pain can cause concern for some surgeons. However, if the surgeon can identify that an injured nerve is the pain generator then there is an opportunity for surgery to greatly improve patients' quality of life. These surgery techniques are well within a hand surgeon's abilities and the need to understand the unique anatomy of each nerve provides a satisfying surgical challenge.

REFERENCES

1. Meyer RA, Raja SN, Campbell JN, et al. Neural activity originating from a neuroma in the baboon. Brain Res 1985;325:255–60.
2. Dellon AL, Mackinnon SE. Susceptibility of the superficial sensory branch of the radial nerve to form painful neuromas. J Hand Surg 1984;9B:42–5.
3. Mackinnon SE, Dellon AL. Overlap of lateral antebrachial cutaneous nerve and superficial sensory branch of the radial nerve. J Hand Surg 1985;10A:522–6.
4. Dellon AL, Mackinnon SE, Pestronk A. Implantation of sensory nerve into muscle: preliminary clinical and experimental observations on neuroma formation. Ann Plast Surg 1984;12:30–40.
5. Mackinnon SE, Dellon AL, Hudson AR, et al. Alteration of neuroma formation by manipulation of neural microenvironment. Plast Reconstr Surg 1985;76:345–52.
6. Dellon AL, Mackinnon SE. Treatment of the painful neuroma by neuroma resection and muscle implantation. Plast Reconstr Surg 1986;77:427–36.
7. Mackinnon SE, Dellon AL. Algorithm for neuroma management. Contemp Orthop 1986;13:15–27.
8. Mackinnon SE, Dellon AL. Pain after radial sensory nerve grafting. J Hand Surg 1986;11B:341–6.
9. Mackinnon SE, Dellon AL. Results of treatment of recurrent dorsoradial wrist neuromas. Ann Plast Surg 1987;19:54–61.
10. Saplys R, Mackinnon SE, Dellon AL. The relationship between nerve entrapment versus neuroma complications and the misdiagnosis of deQuervain's disease. Contemp Orthop 1987;15:51–7.
11. Evans GRD, Dellon AL. Implantation of the palmar cutaneous branch of the median nerve into the pronator quadratus for treatment of painful neuroma. J Hand Surg 1994;19A:203–6.
12. Dellon AL, Aszmann OC. Treatment of dorsal foot neuromas by translocation of nerves into anterolateral compartment. Foot Ankle Int 1998;19:300–3.
13. Wolfort S, Dellon AL. Treatment of recurrent neuroma of the interdigital nerve by neuroma resection and implantation of proximal nerve into muscle in the arch. J Foot Ankle Surg 2001;40:404–10.
14. Kim J, Dellon AL. Neuromas of the calcaneal nerves: diagnosis and treatment. Foot Ankle Int 2001;22:890–4.
15. Kim J, Dellon AL. Tarsal tunnel incisional pain due to neuroma of the posterior branch of saphenous nerve. J Am Podiatr Med Assoc 2001;91:109–13.
16. Dellon AL, Kim J, Ducic I. Painful neuroma of the posterior cutaneous nerve of the forearm after surgery for lateral humeral epicondylitis. J Hand Surg Am 2004;29:387–90.
17. Mackinnon SE, Dellon AL, Hudson AR, et al. Histopathology of compression of the superficial radial nerve in the forearm. J Hand Surg 1986;11A:206–9.
18. Mackinnon SE, Dellon AL, Hudson AR, et al. Chronic human nerve compression: a histologic assessment. Neuropathol Appl Neurobiol 1986;12:547–65.
19. Dellon AL, Andonian E, Rosson GD. CRPS I of the upper or lower extremity: surgical treatment outcomes. J Brachial Plex Peripher Nerve Inj 2009;4:1–15.
20. Buck-Gramcko D. Denervation of the wrist joint. J Hand Surg Am 1977;2:54–61.
21. Dellon AL, Seif SS. Neuroma of the posterior interosseous nerve simulating a recurrent ganglion: case report and anatomical dissection relating the posterior interosseous nerve to the carpus and etiology of dorsal ganglion pain. J Hand Surg 1978;3:326–32.
22. Dellon AL, Mackinnon SE, Daneshvar A. Terminal branch of anterior interosseous nerve as source of wrist pain. J Hand Surg 1984;9B:316–22.
23. Dellon AL. Partial dorsal wrist denervation: resection of distal posterior interosseous nerve. J Hand Surg 1985;10A:527–33.
24. Berger RA. Partial denervation of the wrist: a new approach. Tech Hand Up Extrem Surg 1998;2:25–35.
25. Dellon AL. Partial joint denervation I: wrist, shoulder, elbow. Plast Reconstr Surg 2009;123:197–207.
26. Dellon AL. Partial joint denervation II: knee, ankle. Plast Reconstr Surg 2009;123:208–17.
27. Dellon AL. Partial knee denervation: a review. J Sports Med Doping Stud 2014;4:153.
28. Dellon AL, Ducic I, DeJesus RA. Innervation of the medial humeral epicondyle: implications for medial epicondylar pain. J Hand Surg 2006;31B:331–3.
29. Berry N, Ruccol R, Noumciater MW, et al. Epicondylectomy versus denervation for lateral epicondylitis. Hand (N Y) 2011;6:174–8.
30. Rose N, Forman S, Dellon AL. Denervation of the lateral humeral epicondyle for treatment of chronic lateral humeral epicondylitis. J Hand Surg Am 2013;38:344–9.
31. Laporte D, Hashemi SS, Dellon AL. Sensory innervation of the triangular fibrocartilage: a cadaveric study. J Hand Surg 2014;39:1122–4.
32. Dellon AL. Relief of pitcher's elbow by denervation of the medial humeral epicondyle. J Sports Med Doping Stud 2014;4:135.

33. Lin YT, Berger RA, Berger EJ, et al. Nerve endings of the wrist joint: a preliminary report of the dorsal radiocarpal ligament. J Orthop Res 2006;224: 1225–30.

34. Tomita K, Berger EJ, Berger RA, et al. Distribution of nerve endings in the human dorsal radiocarpal ligament. J Hand Surg Am 2007;32:466–73.

35. Hagert E, Persson JK. Desensitizing the posterior interosseous nerve alters wrist proprioceptive reflexes. J Hand Surg Am 2010;35:1059–66.

36. Gay A, Harbst K, Hansen DK, et al. Effect of partial wrist denervation on wrist kinesthesia: wrist denervation does not impair proprioception. J Hand Surg Am 2011;36:1774–9.

37. Dellon AL, Andronian E, Rosson GD. Lower extremity CRPS: long-term results of surgical treatment of peripheral nerve pain generators. J Foot Ankle Surg 2010;49:33–6.

38. Dellon AL, Mackinnon SE. Radial sensory nerve entrapment. Arch Neurol 1986;43:833–5.

39. Howard M, Lee C, Dellon AL. Documentation of brachial plexus compression (in the thoracic inlet) utilizing provocative neurosensory and muscular testing. J Reconstr Microsurg 2003;19:303–12.

40. Dellon AL. The results of supraclavicular brachial plexus neurolysis (without first rib resection) in management of post-traumatic "thoracic outlet syndrome". J Reconstr Microsurg 1993;9:11–7.

41. Dellon AL. Evaluation of sensibility and re-education of sensation in the hand. 1st edition. Baltimore (MD): Williams and Wilkins; 1981. Available at: Dellon.com.

42. Dellon AL. Somatosensory testing & rehabilitation. Bethesda (MD): American Occupational Medicine Association; 1997.

43. Dellon AL, Mackinnon SE. Injury to the medial antebrachial cutaneous nerve during cubital tunnel surgery. J Hand Surg 1985;10B:33–6.

44. Aszmann OC, Korak KJ, Rab M, et al. Neuroma prevention by end-to-side neurorrhaphy: an experimental study in rats. J Hand Surg Am 2003;28:1022–8.

45. Aszmann OC, Moser V, Frey M. Treatment of painful neuromas via end-to-side neurorrhaphy. Handchir Mikrochir Plast Chir 2010;42:225–32.

46. Mitchell SW. Injuries of nerves and their consequences. Philadelphia: American Academy of Neurology; 1872. p. 179–83. reprint series.

47. Dellon AL. Pain Solutions. chapter 7, RSD. Baltimore (MD): Lightning Source Publishers; 2007. p. 205–31.

The Proper Use of Neurostimulation for Hand Pain

Jason E. Pope, MD[a],*, David Provenzano, MD[b],
Porter McRoberts, MD[c], Timothy Deer, MD[d]

KEYWORDS

- Neuropathic pain • Hand pain • CRPS • Peripheral nerve stimulation • Spinal cord stimulation
- Dorsal root ganglion • Dorsal root ganglion stimulation

KEY POINTS

- Neuropathic pain of the hand can be related to multiple disease processes.
- Neuropathic upper extremity pain disorders include median, radial, and ulnar neuropathy; brachial plexus injuries; complex regional pain syndrome (CRPS) type 1; complex regional pain syndrome type 2 (causalgia); and peripheral neuropathy.
- Neuromodulation is an effective treatment strategy of neuropathic upper extremity pain that has not responded to more conservative measures.
- Neuromodulation therapies include dorsal root ganglion (DRG) spinal stimulation, peripheral nerve stimulation (PNS), and conventional spinal cord stimulation (SCS).
- Physicians should understand when and how to effectively use these therapies.

INTRODUCTION

Upper extremity (UE) neuropathic pain states greatly impact patient functionality and quality of life. Missed workdays associated with complex regional pain syndrome (CRPS) of the UE alone suggest more definitive treatment strategies are necessary.[1] Furthermore, earlier access to advanced pain care therapies may improve outcomes and health care use.[2–4]

This article reviews the evidence on the safety and efficacy data for advanced neuromodulation treatment strategies currently available and surveys future therapies. Therapies covered include spinal cord stimulation (SCS), dorsal root ganglion (DRG) spinal stimulation, and peripheral nerve stimulation (PNS).

Classifications are required for taxonomy purposes. SCS is the placement of electrodes within the neuraxis epidural space with the intent of stimulating the dorsal columns of the spinal cord. DRG spinal stimulation is the placement of leads within the epidural space of the neuraxis with the intent of stimulating the DRG of the spinal cord. PNS is the placement of a lead with the intent of stimulation of peripheral nerves outside of the neuraxis.

Conflicts of Interest: Dr J.E. Pope is a consultant for Medtronic, St. Jude, Flowonix, and Jazz Pharmaceuticals. Dr D. Provenzano is a consultant for Halyard Health, Medtronic, St. Jude Medical, and Trevena. Dr P. McRoberts is a consultant for St. Jude, Medtronic, Flowonix, and SPR therapeutics, and is a minor stockholder in Nevro. Dr T. Deer is a consultant for Bioness, Nevro, Medtronic, St. Jude, Flowonix, and Jazz, and a minor stockholder in Nevro, Bioness, Spinal Therapeutics, and Axonics.
 ^a Summit Pain Alliance, 392 Tesconi Court, Santa Rosa, CA 95401, USA; ^b Pain Diagnostics and Interventional Care, Sewickley, PA 15143, USA; ^c Holy Cross Hospital, Ft Lauderdale, FL 33308, USA; ^d Center for Pain Relief, Charleston, WV 25304, USA
* Corresponding author.
E-mail address: popeje@me.com

These techniques and targets can treat refractory pain when more conservative therapies are inadequate. The world literature of neurostimulation provides insights on how to select the correct patient, therapy, and disease process for intervention. This international experience suggests future directions for the United States. The international perspective is important because many regulatory bodies outside of the United States allow for human investigation of new devices and subsequent approval much earlier than is achieved in the United States. The implanting or referring doctor should consult with their country of practice regarding approvals and availability of devices.

Cause of Neuropathic Pain of the Upper Extremity

The exact prevalence of neuropathy originating from the periphery is unknown, although it is a contributor in the 8% to 10% of the adults with neuropathic pain.[5] There are many neuropathic pain states that affect the UE, including peripheral neuropathy; brachial plexus avulsion injuries; compressive neuropathies of the distal UE; median, ulnar, and radial neuropathy; and CRPS type 1 and type 2.[6,7]

Conservative Treatment Options

Conservative care therapies for UE neuropathic pain syndromes of the hand are focused on the cause of disease. Depending on the type of neuropathic pain, different treatment strategies may be used including physical therapy/occupational therapy, ultrasound (US)-guided injections for diagnostic and therapeutic purposes, surgical intervention, transcutaneous electrical stimulation, nonsteroidal anti-inflammatory drugs, neuropathic pain medications, opioid analgesics, and oral corticosteroids.[8]

NEUROMODULATION OF THE UPPER EXTREMITY

When conservative therapies are inadequate, advanced therapies are used. Neuromodulation techniques have been demonstrated to improve neuropathic pain in the extremity and centrally. These are addressed next in turn.

SPINAL CORD STIMULATION: DORSAL COLUMNS
Background

The clinical use of neurostimulation for the treatment of pain began in the 1960s with the description of the gate-control theory, which posits that nonpainful stimuli can close the "gate" to painful stimuli.[9] Shortly thereafter SCS was introduced by Shealy and coworkers in 1967.[10] Over the last 30 years, important insights and advancements have occurred in the use of SCS for the treatment of multiple pain states and for the modulation of neuropathic, vascular, and visceral pathologic states.[11] Cervical SCS can be used to treat UE pain.

Mechanism of Action

The exact mechanism of action for the SCS on neuropathic pain is still unknown. Initially, Melzack and Wall[9] introduced the gate-control theory and proposed that $A\delta$ and C fibers were inhibited by the activation of $A\beta$.[12] However, other mechanisms may play a significant role, including increasing the dorsal horn inhibitory action of γ-aminobutyric acid, alterations in the activity of wide dynamic range neurons through the orthodomic activation of the primary afferent neurons, activation of the descending inhibitory pain pathways, and modulation of the cholinergic system.[13–16] Furthermore, SCS induces the release of adenosine, serotonin, and norepinephrine.[17–20] In addition to modulating neuropathic pain, SCS has also been shown to assist in the treatment of ischemic pain especially when microcirculatory deficiencies exist.[21–24] Possible mechanisms for SCS to influence peripheral blood flow include (1) modulation of the autonomic nervous system; (2) activation of the descending inhibitory system; and (3) antidromic activation of sensory nerves ($A\delta$ and C fibers), and subsequent release of vasodilator mediators including nitric oxide and calcitonin gene-related peptide.[25–27]

Indications and Patient Selection

Cervical SCS is an effective treatment of neuropathic pain emanating from the neck and UE.[11,28] Pathologic pain states that may respond include cervical radiculopathy, brachial plexus avulsion injuries, CRPS (type 1 and type 2 causalgia), and peripheral neuropathic pain. Patients are selected for SCS after more conservative therapies have proved to be unsuccessful. These treatments include medication management, minimally invasive interventions (eg, stellate ganglion blocks), and occupational and physical therapy. Unfortunately, less than 50% of patients with neuropathic pain find significant improvement in pain control with any pharmacologic drug.[29] Before considering an SCS trial, a patient should undergo a psychological evaluation. Presurgical psychological factors associated with poor outcomes include high levels of somatization, depression, anxiety, and poor coping skills.[30] Other factors that may also negatively influence outcomes include worker compensation and psychological factors, including somatization and catastrophizing behavior.[31,32] Before progressing with an SCS trial the patient's cervical spinal canal diameter should be evaluated.[11,33–36] In addition, optimization of any medical comorbidities including diabetes and tobacco use, which can negatively affect operative outcome, should occur.

Technical Aspects for Both Trial and Implant Stages

In the United States, before implantation of an SCS there must be a trial that demonstrates perceived therapeutic paresthesia overlying the painful area. Initially, patients undergo an SCS trial, which most commonly involves the placement of a cylindrical percutaneous lead through an entry needle into the epidural space. The site of entry is often between T1 and T3 interspaces for neck and UE pain conditions. The lead is advanced into the cervical spine in the posterior epidural space (**Fig. 1**). Mapping of sensory responses to epidural stimulation has demonstrated that UE coverage most often occurs between C2 through C6. The C2-C4 region typically provides shoulder coverage and the C5 and C6 region typically provides hand coverage. The goal of traditional SCS is to provide paresthesia coverage over the painful area. Once the lead is in an appropriate position, adjustments are made in programming parameters including electrode configuration and pulse width, frequency, and amplitude settings. Once the lead is in the appropriate position and configured, a patient trials the SCS system for

approximately 3 to 6 days.[11,37] The lead is then typically removed at the end of the trial, and individuals are asked to evaluate their comfort with the system, pain response, and functional improvement. Predictors of a long-term successful outcome for the SCS trial and implant include the pretrial presence of allodynia and/or hyperalgooia, and functional improvement with trial.[00] Variables most strongly associated with poor SCS outcomes include less than 50% pain relief during the trial and a history of substance abuse.[38] If SCS is being used to modulate peripheral blood flow, transcutaneous oxygen pressure is used to determine if microcirculatory reserves exists that can be effectively modulated by the SCS system.[21]

Individuals that have a successful trial are candidates for the more permanent system and implant. This commonly occurs within 2 to 3 weeks from the trial. During the implantation stage, either a cylindrical percutaneous lead or laminotomy (paddle) leads are placed, with the addition of a surgical placement of an internal pulse generator (IPG), commonly positioned in the low back or infraclavicular area.

Outcomes

Although not studied as frequently as thoracolumbar SCS, cervical SCS has been shown in numerous studies to be associated with improvements in pain control, quality of life indices, and functional improvement. Deer and colleagues[28] demonstrated through an international registry the ability of cervical SCS to improve pain and quality-of-life indices. Patient-reported pain relief

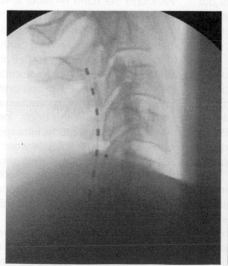
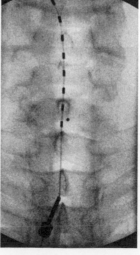

Fig. 1. Percutaneous spinal cord stimulation.

at 12 months postimplantation was 67%. Overall quality of life was reported as improved or greatly improved by 75% of patients at 12 months. The percentage of patients reporting their health had improved or greatly improved was 66% at 12 months. Furthermore, sleep improved with 56% of patients reporting improved or greatly improved sleep patterns at 12 months. Satisfaction scores were also high with cervical SCS with 88% of patients indicating that they were very satisfied or satisfied with their SCS device at 12 months.

Deer and colleagues[28] also completed a systematic literature review on the efficacy of cervical SCS. Twelve studies were identified, which included a total of 211 patients. The 12 studies consisted of four prospective nonrandomized uncontrolled studies, four retrospective studies, and four case series.[24,39–49] Conditions examined in these studies included refractory reflex sympathetic dystrophy (now known as CRPS) and patients with Raynaud disease. Across all the studies, the authors found greater than or equal to 50% pain relief. The two most common adverse events reported were hardware malfunction and lead migration. Complications that may occur include lead migration, lead breakage, abnormal stimulation patterns, and infection.[36]

Specifically for CRPS, SCS has been shown to be an effective treatment.[49–51] When SCS is incorporated into a physical therapy algorithm in comparison with physical therapy alone, SCS has been shown to significantly improve pain scores and global perceived effect.[50,51] SCS has also been shown to improve motor function with documented improvements in grip strength. Pain medication use decreases with cervical SCS. Not only does cervical SCS improve clinical outcomes but it is also more cost-effective than physical therapy alone in the treatment of CRPS and is considered a Grade A technology (ie, compelling evidence for adoption and appropriate use).[52,53]

Case reports have demonstrated successful use of cervical SCS for intractable pain associated with brachial plexus avulsion injuries.[54–56] Intractable pain is highly associated with brachial plexus avulsion injuries and has an incidence of 26% to 90%. Pharmacologic treatment is often unsuccessful,[56] making other alternatives, such as cervical SCS, attractive.

When cervical SCS is used it is important to incorporate this treatment into a multidisciplinary treatment plan that incorporates physical therapy and occupational therapy, medication management, and psychological therapy when appropriate.[57] Cervical SCS should be considered early in the treatment algorithm for UE neuropathic

pain conditions that have not improved with more conservative measures.[32,58]

In addition to the ability to improve pain control, cervical SCS has also been associated with changes in vascular flow to the affected extremity. SCS has shown improvement in Raynaud disease. Furthermore, cervical SCS has been shown to improve wound healing and increase blood supply in individuals with arterial steel syndrome.[59] SCS can represent an additional tool for these challenging vascular patients.

Traditional SCS for pain relies on the need for perceived therapeutic paresthesia overlying the painful area.[60] Even with the defined success of traditional SCS, recent data suggest that novel waveforms may have the ability to improve and augment traditional therapy. New waveforms being studied that have shown significant promise for other neuropathic pain states (eg, lower extremity radicular symptoms) include high-frequency 10-kHz SCS and burst stimulation.[61,62] A case report described burst stimulation salvage for diminishing coverage with traditional SCS in a patient with left UE CRPS.[63] More prospective, higher-powered studies are needed to determine the placement of novel waveform strategies in the treatment algorithm for UE neuropathic pain.

As neuromodulation techniques advance, so does refinement in the technology and strategy. Future directions include limiting the positionality of stimulation patterns, improving patient selection, and further work to limit biologic- and hardware-related complications.

DORSAL ROOT GANGLION SPINAL STIMULATION

Although the hand projects a wide bandwidth of neural feedback to the cervical spine, stimulation of specific and isolated subcomponents of the hand can be challenging with traditional SCS (Fig. 2). Holsheimer and Barolat[64] examined 3897 bipolar and unipolar combinations from 106 patients and yielded a comprehensive series of likelihood ratios for paresthesia generation (and thus pain relief) in the body, including the hand. At the time of their study, intraspinal neuromodulation stimulation techniques were limited to the dorsal columns and dorsal root entry zone ablations. Techniques to specifically stimulate the DRG had not been developed. They found that stimulation of the C1-2 to T2 cord yielded a 60% to 75% probability of stimulating either the radial forearm or median hand.[64] The ulnar hand was served by the cord at C5-T1 60% to 75% of the time.[64]

Although traditional SCS can improve pain, function, and medication use for patients with

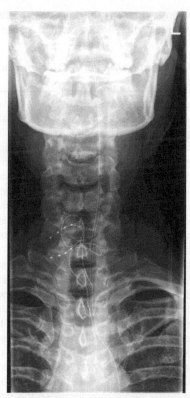

Fig. 2. Cervical DRG stimulation placement.

neuropathic pain, DRG spinal stimulation offers an opportunity to refine the treatment of hand and UE pain. The DRG refinements could include more specific dermatographic stimulation, with less variability in coverage location and intensity. This is a key improvement. An advantage of the DRG target nerves is that they move little because the DRG is a relatively fixed structure within the spine and there is little bathing cerebrospinal fluid. The DRG plays a vital role in the transmission and reinforcement of chronic pain. It has been extensively shown in neuropathic pain to express abnormal, spontaneous activity.[65–67] DRG stimulation requires a preoperative evaluation of the target neuroforaminal space, with a specific inspection for pre-existing scar tissue and other anatomic variants of the area of intended implant.

Although there are no large, prospective studies for the use of cervical DRG stimulation, several case reports exist. In a retrospective review presented at the North American Neuromodulation Society 17th Annual meeting, cervical DRG stimulation yielded 66% improvement at 3 months on perceived chronic hand pain secondary to amputation. In a separate patient from the same report, cervical DRG stimulation yielded 51%

improvement in hand pain from cervical trauma.[68] Another case presented was cervical DRG stimulation for severe hand pain as a function of brachial plexus avulsion yielding 89% and 94% reduction of C7 and C8 mediated hand pain at 1 week and 12 weeks, respectively.[69] A separate report was presented of a patient who presented with glove-type hand pain failing T2 sympathetic block, conventional SCS, and high-frequency stimulation; ultimately DRG trial stimulation of C7 and C8 provided 35% to 40% relief.[70] Other recent case reports have presented cervical C7 DRG stimulation to treat chronic radial nerve injury pain yielding a reduction in visual analog scale (VAS) from 70 at baseline to 20 at 6-month follow-up.[71] Additionally reported was a pooled data presentation of 19 subjects with CRPS of the upper limb treated with DRG stimulation revealing a drop for an average VAS at baseline of 82 to 30 at 6 months.[72]

Future work is warranted and needed on the applicability of DRG cervical stimulation for the treatment of UE hand pain. Initial case reports are encouraging with regards to efficacy and safety, although validation of this research is needed through large prospective observational and randomized controlled studies.

PERIPHERAL NERVE STIMULATION

PNS strategies are useful in the treatment of neuropathic pain of the hand following peripheral nerve injury. These neuropathic pain states can be from distal and/or proximal nerve injuries. Traditionally, PNS therapies were performed as an open surgical procedure with dissection to the nerve, fascial grafting, and open lead placement. This more invasive approach can lead to substantial scarring around the nerve.[73,74] New techniques were introduced to reduce the morbidity of the open procedure, in some cases using US as a means to help identify the nerve. Similarly, nerve localization by stimulation strategies, as used in the regional anesthesia for perioperative nerve blocks for postoperative pain, may offer another tool to place PNS.[75]

PNS is an attractive option because it focuses on the injured nerve pathway outside of the spinal cord. However there are clear challenges with peripheral nerve interventions. The primary barrier to PNS is the equipment. Current equipment is designed for the neuraxis, necessitating modification for use in the periphery.[75] Challenges for using PNS in the distal UE include leads crossing joints and limited locations for IPG placement.[76] Currently these equipment issues still limit the full use of PNS in the distal upper limb.

Spinal Cord Stimulation Equipment in the Periphery

Identified targets for PNS to cover pain in the hand often focus on the brachial plexus.[77] Anatomically, the peripheral nerves most commonly targeted are the ulnar, radial, and median. Huntoon and Burgher[78] described techniques for PNS with US guidance, and open techniques have also been described and are discussed in order.[79]

Ultrasound-Guided Percutaneous Lead Placement Technique

The ulnar nerve is identified at the medial epicondyle and traced proximally to its location where it descends medially to the brachial artery, anterior to the triceps, with the US probe in the axial orientation. The median nerve is located by placement of the probe in the transverse orientation and scanned distally from the elbow to a site near the antecubital fossa at the level of the pronater teres heads.[78] The radial nerve is located as it runs near the humerus, laterally approximately 10 to 14 cm proximal to the lateral epicondyle.[78] Although these techniques have been described, implantation of the IPG limits applicability for everyday use. In addition lead migration limits technical success.

Open Peripheral Nerve Paddle Lead Placement Stimulation

Peripheral nerve paddle stimulation is performed with open dissection to the named nerve and placement of an electrode. The epineurium of the nerve is identified and dissected, allowing for paddle lead placement.[79,80] Because this technique requires manipulation of the nerve, general anesthesia is suggested. There is long-term follow-up of patients treated with paddle PNS for UE neuropathic pain. These patients were treated for either median or ulnar neuropathy and were followed[79] over 20 years and had durable relief. PNS paddle technique seems to offer long-term efficacy in

some patients. However, invasiveness of the technique and equipment issues has led to low use.

Innovative Peripheral Nerve Stimulation–Specific Systems

New technologies have entered into the market with the interest of helping solve the challenges previously mentioned, with equipment crafted specifically for use in the periphery. These technologies may offer advancements in PNS, and include the minimally invasive SmartPatch and MicroPulse Technologies by SPR Therapeutics (Cleveland, OH). Recently a randomized prospective study led to Food and Drug Administration approval of a novel PNS device (Stimrouter, Bioness, Vallencia, CA).[81]

The SmartPatch technology by SPR uses a fine-wire electrode with an anchoring barb and electrode (**Fig. 3**). This lead is placed under US guidance through a 20-gauge needle with correct placement confirmed with paresthesias. The system is used with an implantable IPG or an external device, depending on indication and use of therapy. These devices work under the principle that increasing the electrode distance (0.5–3.0 cm) from the target nerve may increase the threshold of nontarget fibers and allow for selective stimulation of the target fibers, widening the therapeutic window within the nerve.[82,83] Rauck and colleagues[83] reported on a feasibility study looking at the ability for the SPR device to treat postamputation pain of the lower extremity with remote stimulation (0.5–3 cm away from target nerve). There were 16 subjects who had stimulation of the femoral and/or the sciatic nerve. In this prospective study, nine were qualified as responders following 2-week therapy of greater than 30% pain score reduction and improvement in quality of life in a self-reported measure.

The Bioness StimRouter System was designed to treat pain of the trunk and extremities, specifically peripheral nerve mononeuropathies (**Fig. 4**).

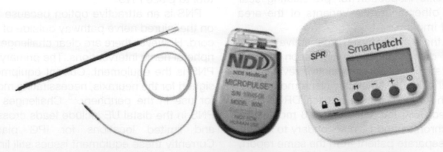

Fig. 3. SPR smart patch. (*Courtesy of* SPR Therapeutics, LLC, Cleveland, OH; with permission.)

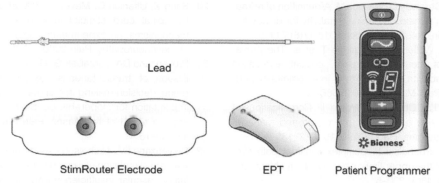

Fig. 4. Bioness stimRouter system. (*Courtesy of* Bioness Inc, Valencia, CA; with permission.)

The StimRouter system consists of a lead containing a receiver and three electrodes for stimulation. The lead has a silicon anchor that holds the lead in place. The external pulse generator is placed over the skin and transmits radiofrequency signal to generate electrical stimulation wirelessly. After feasibility studies,[84] a prospective, multicenter, randomized, double-blinded, partial crossover study powered to detect safety and efficacy was performed. The patients were randomized after implantation to either the control arm of no stimulation or the experimental arm consisting of stimulation, with follow-up for 3 months, after which time the control arm was allowed to crossover. The primary end point was safety and pain relief defined as greater than 30% of pain reduction with no escalation of pain medicine. A total of 38% percent of the stimulation group achieved the primary end point, with no adverse events reported in either arm. None of the other peripheral systems discussed in this section has this level of evidence.

Table 1
Evidence assessment of neuromodulation strategies for the hand

Neuromodulation Strategy	Evidence Level[a]	Strength Grade
Cervical SCS	I	A
PNS	II-2	B
DRG spinal stimulation	III	I

[a] US Prevention Services Task Force criteria.
Data from Guayatt GH, Sackett DL, Sinclair JC, et al. Users' guides to the medical literature: IX. A method for grading health care recommendations. JAMA 1995;274:1800–4; and Harris RP, Helfand M, Woolf SH, et al; Methods Work Group; Third US Prevention Service Task Force. Current methods of the US Preventive Services Task Force: a review of the process. Am J Prev Med 2001;20:21–35.

SUMMARY

Neuropathic pain of the hand can be a debilitating condition, stemming from multiple causes. When simple conservative therapy fails, neuromodulation can play an integral role in treatment success. Of the neuromodulation therapies mentioned, varying levels of evidence exist. Using the US Prevention Services Task Force criteria for evidence synthesis and guidance in determining their strength, recommendations can be drawn.[85,86] The grade of strength for using these neuromodulation therapies to treat neuropathic pain of the hand is listed in **Table 1**.

These evidence-based approaches include traditional SCS, PNS, and DRG spinal stimulation in some non–United States pain markets. As can be appreciated, cervical SCS has Level I evidence and a Grade A recommendation to treat neuropathic pain of the hand related to CRPS. The StimRuter Bioness Device has Level I evidence to treat mononeuropathies of the hand. As these therapies continue to evolve, so to will their placement within the pain care algorithm, grounded by a foundation of evidence to improve patient safety and management of these patients with difficult neuropathic pain.

REFERENCES

1. Stanton-Hicks M. Complex regional pain syndrome: manifestations and the role of neuromodulation in its management. J Pain Symptom Manage 2006;31(4 Suppl):S20–4.
2. Porree L, Krames E, Pope J, et al. Spinal cord stimulation as treatment for complex regional pain syndrome should be considered earlier than last resort therapy. Neuromodulation 2013;16(2):125–41.
3. Kumar K, Toth C, Nath RK, et al. Epidrual spinal cord stimulation for treatment of chronic pain—some predictors of success. A 15 year experience. Surg Neurol 1998;2:110–20.

4. Deer T, Caraway D, Wallace M. A definition of refractory pain to help determine suitability for device implantation. Neuromodulation 2014;17(8):711–5.

5. Yawn B, Wollan P, Weingarten T, et al. The prevalence of neuropathic pain: clinical evaluation compared with screening tools in a community population. Pain Med 2009;10(3):586–93.

6. Santosa KB, Chung KC, Waljee JF. Complications of compressive neuropathy: prevention and management strategies. Hand Clin 2015;31(2):139–49.

7. Żyluk A, Puchalski P. Complex regional pain syndrome of the upper limb: a review. Neurol Neurochir Pol 2014;48(3):200–5.

8. Atalay NS, Ercidogan O, Akkaya N. Prednisolone in complex regional pain syndrome. Pain Physician 2014;17:179–85.

9. Melzack R, Wall PD. Pain mechanisms: a new theory. Science 1965;150:971–9.

10. Shealy CN, Taslitz N, Mortimer JT, et al. Electrical inhibition of pain: experimental evaluation. Anesth Analg 1967;46:299–305.

11. Deer TR, Mekhail N, Provenzano D, et al. The appropriate use of neurostimulation of the spinal cord and peripheral nervous system for the treatment of chronic pain and ischemic diseases: the neuromodulation appropriateness consensus committee. Neuromodulation 2014;17:515–50.

12. Stojanovic MP, Abdi S. Spinal cord stimulation. Pain Physician 2002;5:156–66.

13. Cui JG, O'Connor WT, Ungerstedt U, et al. Spinal cord stimulation attenuates augmented dorsal horn release of excitatory amino acids in mononeuropathy via a GABAergic mechanism. Pain 1997;73: 87–95.

14. Meyerson BA, Cui JG, Yakhnitsa V, et al. Modulation of spinal pain mechanisms by spinal cord stimulation and the potential role of adjuvant pharmacotherapy. Stereotact Funct Neurosurg 1997;68: 129–40.

15. Schechtmann G, Song Z, Ultenius C, et al. Cholinergic mechanisms involved in the pain relieving effect of spinal cord stimulation in a model of neuropathy. Pain 2008;139:136–45.

16. Yakhnitsa V, Linderoth B, Meyerson BA. Spinal cord stimulation attenuates dorsal horn neuronal hyperexcitability in a rat model of mononeuropathy. Pain 1999;79:223–33.

17. Cui JG, Sollevi A, Linderoth B, et al. Adenosine receptor activation suppresses tactile hypersensitivity and potentiates spinal cord stimulation in mononeuropathic rats. Neurosci Lett 1997;223:173–6.

18. Foreman RD, Linderoth B. Neural mechanisms of spinal cord stimulation. Int Rev Neurobiol 2012; 107:87–119.

19. Meyerson BA, Linderoth B. Mechanisms of spinal cord stimulation in neuropathic pain. Neurol Res 2000;22:285–92.

20. Song Z, Ultenius C, Meyerson BA, et al. Pain relief by spinal cord stimulation involves serotonergic mechanisms: an experimental study in a rat model of mononeuropathy. Pain 2009;147:241–8.

21. Provenzano DA, Jarzabek G, Georgevich P. The utilization of transcutaneous oxygen pressures to guide decision-making for spinal cord stimulation implantation for inoperable peripheral vascular disease: a report of two cases. Pain Physician 2008; 11:909–16.

22. Provenzano DA, Nicholson L, Jarzabek G, et al. Spinal cord stimulation utilization to treat the microcirculatory vascular insufficiency and ulcers associated with scleroderma: a case report and review of the literature. Pain Med 2011;12:1331–5.

23. Neuhauser B, Perkmann R, Klingler PJ, et al. Clinical and objective data on spinal cord stimulation for the treatment of severe Raynaud's phenomenon. Am Surg 2001;67:1096–7.

24. Francaviglia N, Silvestro C, Maiello M, et al. Spinal cord stimulation for the treatment of progressive systemic sclerosis and Raynaud's syndrome. Br J Neurosurg 1994;8:567–71.

25. Tanaka S, Barron KW, Chandler MJ, et al. Role of primary afferents in spinal cord stimulation-induced vasodilation: characterization of fiber types. Brain Res 2003;959:191–8.

26. Tanaka S, Barron KW, Chandler MJ, et al. Low intensity spinal cord stimulation may induce cutaneous vasodilation via CGRP release. Brain Res 2001; 896:183–7.

27. Wu M, Linderoth B, Foreman RD. Putative mechanisms behind effects of spinal cord stimulation on vascular diseases: a review of experimental studies. Auton Neurosci 2008;138:9–23.

28. Deer TR, Skaribas IM, Haider N, et al. Effectiveness of cervical spinal cord stimulation for the management of chronic pain. Neuromodulation 2014;17: 265–71 [discussion: 271].

29. Dworkin RH, Backonja M, Rowbotham MC, et al. Advances in neuropathic pain: diagnosis, mechanisms, and treatment recommendations. Arch Neurol 2003;60:1524–34.

30. Celestin J, Edwards RR, Jamison RN. Pretreatment psychosocial variables as predictors of outcomes following lumbar surgery and spinal cord stimulation: a systematic review and literature synthesis. Pain Med 2009;10:639–53.

31. Kumar K, Wilson JR, Taylor RS, et al. Complications of spinal cord stimulation, suggestions to improve outcome, and financial impact. J Neurosurg 2006; 5:191–203.

32. Kumar K, Caraway DL, Rizvi S, et al. Current challenges in spinal cord stimulation. Neuromodulation 2014;17(Suppl 1):22–35.

33. Narouze S, Benzon HT, Provenzano DA, et al. Interventional spine and pain procedures in patients on

antiplatelet and anticoagulant medications: guidelines from the American Society of Regional Anesthesia and Pain Medicine, the European Society of Regional Anaesthesia and Pain Therapy, the American Academy of Pain Medicine, the International Neuromodulation Society, the North American Neuromodulation Society, and the World Institute of Pain. Reg Anesth Pain Med 2015;40:182–212.

34. Deer TR, Thomson S, Pope JE, et al. International neuromodulation society critical assessment: guideline review of implantable neurostimulation devices. Neuromodulation 2014;17(7):678–85.

35. Deer TR, Krames E, Mekhail N, et al. The appropriate use of neurostimulation: new and evolving neurostimulation therapies and applicable treatment for chronic pain and selected disease States. Neuromodulation 2014;17:599–615.

36. Deer TR, Mekhail N, Provenzano D, et al. The appropriate use of neurostimulation: avoidance and treatment of complications of neurostimulation therapies for the treatment of chronic pain. Neuromodulation 2014;17:571–98.

37. Chincholkar M, Eldabe S, Strachan R, et al. Prospective analysis of the trial period for spinal cord stimulation treatment for chronic pain. Neuromodulation 2011;14:523–8 [discussion: 528–9].

38. Williams KA, Gonzalez-Fernandez M, Hamzehzadeh S, et al. A multi-center analysis evaluating factors associated with spinal cord stimulation outcome in chronic pain patients. Pain Med 2011;12:1142–53.

39. Calvillo O, Racz G, Didie J, et al. Neuroaugmentation in the treatment of complex regional pain syndrome of the upper extremity. Acta Orthop Belg 1998;64:57–63.

40. Simpson BA, Bassett G, Davies K, et al. Cervical spinal cord stimulation for pain: a report on 41 patients. Neuromodulation 2003;6:20–6.

41. Whitworth LA, Feler CA. C1-C2 sublaminar insertion of paddle leads for the management of chronic painful conditions of the upper extremity. Neuromodulation 2003;6:153–7.

42. Kumar K, Rizvi S, Bnurs SB. Spinal cord stimulation is effective in management of complex regional pain syndrome I: fact or fiction. Neurosurgery 2011;69: 566–78 [discussion: 578–80].

43. Wolter T, Kieselbach K. Cervical spinal cord stimulation; an analysis of 20 patients with long-term follow-up. Pain Physician 2012;15:203–12.

44. Robaina FJ, Dominguez M, Diaz M, et al. Spinal cord stimulation for relief of chronic pain in vasospastic disorders of the upper limbs. Neurosurgery 1989; 24:63–7.

45. Vallejo R, Kramer J, Benyamin R. Neuromodulation of the cervical spinal cord in the treatment of chronic intractable neck and upper extremity pain: a case series and review of the literature. Pain Physician 2007;10:305–11.

46. Hayek SM, Veizi IE, Stanton-Hicks M. Four-limb neurostimulation with neuroelectrodes placed in the lower cervical epidural space. Anesthesiology 2009;110:681–4.

47. Moens M, De Smedt A, Brouns R, et al. Retrograde C0-C1 insertion of cervical plate electrode for chronic intractable neck and arm pain. World Neurosurg 2011;76:352–4 [discussion: 268–9].

48. Wolter I, Winkelmuller M. Continuous versus intermittent spinal cord stimulation: an analysis of factors influencing clinical efficacy. Neuromodulation 2012; 15:13–9 [discussion: 20].

49. Forouzanfar T, Kemler MA, Weber WE, et al. Spinal cord stimulation in complex regional pain syndrome: cervical and lumbar devices are comparably effective. Br J Anaesth 2004;92:348–53.

50. Kemler MA, Barendse GA, van Kleef M, et al. Spinal cord stimulation in patients with chronic reflex sympathetic dystrophy. N Engl J Med 2000;343:618–24.

51. Kemler MA, De Vet HC, Barendse GA, et al. The effect of spinal cord stimulation in patients with chronic reflex sympathetic dystrophy: two years' follow-up of the randomized controlled trial. Ann Neurol 2004;55:13–8.

52. Kemler MA, Furnee CA. Economic evaluation of spinal cord stimulation for chronic reflex sympathetic dystrophy. Neurology 2002;59:1203–9.

53. Kemler MA, Raphael JH, Bentley A, et al. The cost-effectiveness of spinal cord stimulation for complex regional pain syndrome. Value Health 2010;13: 735–42.

54. Abdel-Aziz S, Ghaleb AH. Cervical spinal cord stimulation for the management of pain from brachial plexus avulsion. Pain Med 2014;15:712–4.

55. Chang Chien GC, Candido KD, Saeed K, et al. Cervical spinal cord stimulation treatment of deafferentation pain from brachial plexus avulsion injury complicated by complex regional pain syndrome. A Case Rep 2014;3:29–34.

56. Lai HY, Lee CY, Lee ST. High cervical spinal cord stimulation after failed dorsal root entry zone surgery for brachial plexus avulsion pain. Surg Neurol 2009; 72:286–9 [discussion: 289].

57. Stanton-Hicks MD, Burton AW, Bruehl SP, et al. An updated interdisciplinary clinical pathway for CRPS: report of an expert panel. Pain Pract 2002;2:1–16.

58. Rizvi S, Kumar K. Spinal cord stimulation for chronic pain: the importance of early referral. Pain Manag 2014;4:329–31.

59. De Caridi G, Massara M, Benedetto F, et al. Adjuvant spinal cord stimulation improves wound healing of peripheral tissue loss due to steal syndrome of the hand: clinical challenge treating a difficult case. Int Wound J 2014. [Epub ahead of print].

60. Pope JE, Falowski S, Deer TR. Advanced waveforms and frequency with spinal cord stimulation. Expert Rev Med Devices 2015;12(4):431–7.

61. Kapural L. SENZA Study: Multicenter Randomized Controlled Study Comparing HF10 to SCSf for low back and leg pain. Presented at NANS. Los Vegas, NV, December, 2014.

62. De Vos CC, Bom MJ, Vanneste S, et al. Burst spinal cord stimulation evaluated in patients with failed back surgery syndrome and painful diabetic neuropathy. Neuromodulation 2014;17(2):152–9.

63. Kriek N, Groenewg G, Huygen FJ. Burst spinal cord stimulation in a patient with complex regional pain syndrome: a 2-year follow-up. Pain Pract 2015; 15(6):E59–64.

64. Holsheimer J, Barolat G. Spinal geometry and paresthesia coverage in spinal cord stimulation. Neuromodulation 1998;1(3):129–36.

65. Wang W, Gu J, Li YQ, et al. Are voltage-gated sodium channels on the dorsal root ganglion involved in the development of neuropathic pain? Mol Pain 2011;7:16.

66. Sapunar D, Ljubkovic M, Lirk P, et al. Distinct membrane effects of spinal nerve ligation on injured and adjacent dorsal root ganglion neurons in rats. Anesthesiology 2005;103(2):360–76.

67. Xie WR, Deng H, Li H, et al. Robust increase of cutaneous sensitivity, cytokine production and sympathetic sprouting in rats with localized inflammatory irritation of the spinal ganglia. Neuroscience 2006; 142(3):809–22.

68. Wahlstedt A, Leljevahl E. Spinal cord stimulation of the dorsal root ganglion for post surgical pain. Poster: North America Neuromodulation Society Meeting. Los Vegas, NV, December, 2013.

69. Thoma R, Neumann H, Smet I, et al. Pathophysiology of brachial plexus lesion and the role of dorsal root ganglion in modulation of pain. Poster: North America Neuromodulation Society Meeting. Los Vegas, NV, December, 2013.

70. Mitchell B. Dorsal root ganglion stimulation for neuropathic dysaesthesia: A case report. Poster: North America Neuromodulation Society Meeting. Los Vegas, NV, December, 2013.

71. Francois E, Vanderick B. Dorsal root ganglion as a target for treatment of neuropathy of radial nerve through targeted spinal cord stimulation. Poster: North America Neuromodulation Society Meeting. Los Vegas, NV, December, 2014.

72. Huygen FJ, Barabidharan G, Simpson K, et al. An upper limb neuropathic pain cohort treated with stimulation of dorsal root ganglia: pooled data from four prospective European studies. Poster: North America Neuromodulation Society Meeting. Los Vegas, NV, December, 2014.

73. Hassenusch SJ, Stanton-Hicks M, Schoppa D, et al. Long-term results of peripheral nerve stimulation for reflex sympathetic dystrophy. J Neurosurg 1996; 84(3):415–23.

74. Stanton-Hicks M, Salamon J. Stimulation of the central and peripheral nervous system for the control of pain. J Clin Neurophysiol 1997;14(1):46–62.

75. Slavin KV. Technical aspects of peripheral nerve stimulation: hardware and complications. Prog Neurol Surg 2011;24:189–202.

76. Deer TR, Pope JE, Kaplan M. A novel method of neurostimulation of the peripheral nervous system: the StimRouter implantable device. Pain Manag 2012;16(2):113–7.

77. Van De Velde J, Wouters J, Vercauteren T, et al. Morphometric atlas selection for automatic brachial plexus segmentation. Int J Radiat Oncol Biol Phys 2015;92(3):691–8.

78. Huntoon MA, Burgher AH. Ultrasound-guided permanent implantation of peripheral nerve stimulation (PNS) system for neuropathic pain of the extremities: original cases and outcomes. Pain Med 2009;10: 1369–77.

79. Kupers R, Laere KV, Calenbergh FV, et al. Multimodal therapeutic assessment of peripheral nerve stimulation in neuropathic pain: five case reports with a 20-year follow-up. Eur J Pain 2011;15:161. e1–9.

80. Gofeld M, Hanlon JG. Ultrasound-guided placement of a paddle lead onto peripheral nerves: surgical anatomy and methodology. Neuromodulation 2014; 17:48–53.

81. Available at: https://clinicaltrials.gov/ct2/show/ NCT00665132?term=stimrouter&rank=1. Accessed April, 2015.

82. Rauck RL, Kapural L, Cohen SP, et al. Peripheral nerve stimulation for the treatment of postamputation pain: a case report. Pain Pract 2012;12:649–55.

83. Rauck RL, Cohen SP, Gilmore CA, et al. Treatment of post-amputation pain with peripheral nerve stimulation. Neuromodulation 2014;17:188–97.

84. Deer TR, Levy RM, Rosenfeld EL. Prospective clinical study of a new implantable peripheral nerve stimulation device to treat chronic pain. Clin J Pain 2010;26(5):359–72.

85. Guayatt GH, Sackett DL, Sinclair JC, et al. Users' guides to the medical literature: IX. A method for grading health care recommendations. JAMA 1995;274:1800–4.

86. Harris RP, Helfand M, Woolf SH, et al, Methods Work Group, Third US Prevention Service Task Force. Current methods of the US Preventive Services Task Force: a review of the process. Am J Prev Med 2001;20:21–35.

Future Directions for Pain Management
Lessons from the Institute of Medicine Pain Report and the National Pain Strategy

Sean Mackey, MD, PhD*

KEYWORDS

- Precision medicine • Learning health systems • National Pain Strategy • Chronic pain
- Institute of Medicine

KEY POINTS

- Chronic pain affects 100 million Americans and costs our country half a trillion dollars per year.
- Chronic pain can be a disease in itself. We need to better understand the complex mechanisms of pain and translate these mechanisms into safe and effective therapies.
- We need to increase and incentivize the use of interdisciplinary, team-based assessment of chronic pain, particularly in complex cases.
- For a precision pain medicine approach, we need improved data that characterizes the individual pain experience and the outcomes of treatments.

INTRODUCTION

Perioperative and chronic pain management has advanced significantly during the past several decades. We are moving beyond the Cartesian notion of pain in which stimulus or injury is directly related to pain. Instead, we have learned that pain is a uniquely individual and subjective experience that involves not only biological but also psychological and social factors. **Fig. 1** illustrates the multidimensional nature of the pain experience.

Our increasing knowledge of the mechanisms and factors related to the multidimensional nature of pain has translated into improved understanding of the care for the patient in pain. We have improved surgeries, interventional procedures, medications, psychologic interventions, physical therapy, and complementary approaches. We also have greater appreciation for the need for an interdisciplinary, team-based approach to optimize pain care, particularly for more complex cases. This increase in our treatment approaches is particularly important in light of our country's current prescription opioid epidemic. In fact, opioids are continuing to be moved down the list of approaches as more efficacious treatments are identified and the deleterious effects of opioids on some patients better appreciated.

Despite these advances, we still have millions of people suffering from pain with a cost in the billions to society. Where do we go from here? Two recently released national publications outline a clear path forward for the future of pain assessment, prevention, management, and research. The first of these, the *Relieving Pain In America: A Blueprint for Transforming Prevention, Care, Education, and Research* report from the Institute of Medicine (IOM), provides the vision and high-level view of

The author has nothing to disclose.
Departments of Anesthesiology, Perioperative and Pain Medicine, Neurosciences and Neurology, Stanford University School of Medicine, Palo Alto, CA 94304, USA
* Stanford University, 1070 Arastradero, Suite 200, Palo Alto, CA 94304.
E-mail address: smackey@stanford.edu

Hand Clin 32 (2016) 91–98
http://dx.doi.org/10.1016/j.hcl.2015.08.012
0749-0712/16/$ – see front matter © 2016 Elsevier Inc. All rights reserved.

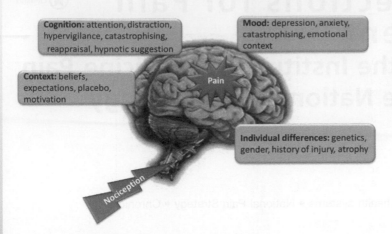

Fig. 1. Multidimensional aspects of pain. Pain is an integrative sum of nociceptive input (ie, signals from periphery during injury or surgery) combined with multiple factors that modulate this input to generate the complex and individual experience of pain.

the path forward. The second, the *National Pain Strategy* (NPS), shows us how to achieve the vision of optimal pain assessment, prevention, and care. This discussion emphasizes information relevant for the readers of this journal.

Relieving Pain in America: a Blueprint for Transforming Prevention, Care, Education, and Research

As part of the 2010 Patient Protection and Affordable Care Act, the IOM was charged "to increase the recognition of pain as a significant public health problem in the United States." Accordingly, Department of Health and Human Services (HHS), through the National Institutes of Health (NIH), requested that the IOM conduct a study to assess the state of the science regarding pain research, care, and education and to make recommendations to advance the field. The efforts of the multidisciplinary committee that was formed, in which I was honored to be a member, resulted in the IOM report, *Relieving Pain in America*. This report was guided by several underlying principles noted in **Box 1**.

One of the charges to the IOM Pain Committee was to "review and quantify the public health significance of pain." We commissioned an econometric study that estimated that an astounding 100 million American adults are affected by chronic pain, exceeding the numbers of those affected by diabetes, cancer, and heart disease combined.[1] These estimates of chronic pain are an overall underestimate because they do not include adults affected by acute pain, children with either acute or chronic pain, or adults living in long-term care facilities, in the military, or in prison.[2] Furthermore, pain affects millions of Americans throughout their lifetime, increases

disability, consumes resources in the health care system, and results in a significant economic burden for the entire nation. The staggering socioeconomic burden of pain is thought to exceed half a trillion dollars per year. Overall, chronic pain has significant effects on the individual in relation to physical functioning, quality of life, and psychological well-being.

To address the problem of pain, we put forward that our nation should adopt a population-level prevention and management strategy and tasked HHS with developing a comprehensive plan with specific goals, actions, stakeholders, and timeframes. This plan should:

- Heighten awareness about pain and its health consequences
- Emphasize the prevention of pain
- Improve pain assessment and management in the delivery of health care and financing programs of the federal government
- Use public health communication strategies to inform patients on how to manage their own pain
- Address disparities in the experience of pain among subgroups of Americans.

One of the key messages was that better data on pain are needed, including data on pain prevalence, incidence, and treatments. This includes data on characteristics of both acute and chronic pain, as well as factors that cause pain after surgery to develop into chronic pain. We are only starting to better understand the factors that lead patients to develop persistent postsurgical pain and persistent use of opioids.[3–5] Much of that knowledge points to factors that patients bring to the operating room (eg, catastrophizing, early adverse life events, depression, anxiety) or an

---

Box 1
Relieving pain in America: underlying principles guiding the IOM committee

- A moral imperative: Effective pain management is a moral imperative, a professional responsibility, and the duty of people in the healing professions.
- Chronic pain can be a disease in itself: Chronic pain has a distinct pathologic effect, causing changes throughout the nervous system that often worsen over time. It has significant psychological and cognitive correlates and can constitute a serious, separate disease entity.
- Value of comprehensive treatment. Pain results from a combination of biological, psychological, and social factors and often requires comprehensive approaches to prevention and management.
- Need for interdisciplinary approaches: Given chronic pain's diverse effects, interdisciplinary assessment and treatment may produce the best results for people with the most severe and persistent pain problems.
- Importance of prevention: Chronic pain has such severe impacts on all aspects of the lives of its sufferers that every effort should be made to achieve both primary prevention (eg, in surgery for broken hip) and secondary prevention (of the transition from the acute to the chronic state) through early intervention.
- Wider use of existing knowledge: Although there is much more to be learned about pain and its treatment, even existing knowledge is not always used effectively, and thus substantial numbers of people suffer unnecessarily.
- The conundrum of opioids: The committee recognizes the serious problem of diversion and abuse of opioid drugs, as well as questions about their usefulness long-term, but believes that when opioids are used as prescribed and appropriately monitored, they can be safe and effective, especially for acute, postoperative, and procedural pain, as well as for patients near the end of life who desire more pain relief.
- Roles for patients and clinicians: The effectiveness of pain treatments depends greatly on the strength of the clinician-patient relationship; pain treatment is never about the clinician's intervention alone, but about the clinician and patient (and family) working together.
- Value of a public health and community-based approach: Many features of the problem of pain lend themselves to public health approaches, including a concern about the large number of people affected, disparities in occurrence and treatment, and the goal of prevention cited above. Public health education can help counter the myths, misunderstandings, stereotypes, and stigma that hinder better care.

From Institute of Medicine (U.S.). Committee on Advancing Pain Research Care and Education. Relieving pain in America : a blueprint for transforming prevention, care, education, and research. Washington, D.C.: National Academies Press; 2011. *Reprinted with permission from* the National Academies Press, Copyright © 2011 National Academy of Sciences.

---

injury that contributes significantly to the development of persistent pain and opioid use. The IOM report also called for increased efforts on preventative measures that will reduce the incidence of persistent pain after surgery and injury.

The IOM report also called for tailoring pain care to each person's experience with an emphasis on self-management if possible. Coordinated, interdisciplinary pain assessment and care for patients with complex pain should be better incentivized financially and promoted. Furthermore, education for both persons with pain and those who provide pain care needs to be enhanced. The IOM report called for a redesign of educational programs to foster an understanding of the complex biological and psychosocial aspects of pain and the multimodal approach to treatment. This redesign of

pain curriculum crosses all medical specialties, including surgery, medicine, physical and occupational therapy, nursing, and all other groups that care for the person in pain. In addition, although we called for increased research on the mechanisms responsible for pain and for the development of safe and effective treatments, we also recognized that there is a wealth of existing knowledge. We must ensure that this knowledge is transmitted to people suffering from pain and to the providers who care for them.

Finally, the IOM committee noted that research has made remarkable gains in characterizing the biological, cognitive, and psychological mechanisms of pain, and the future promises advances in several fields, from genomic and cellular through behavioral mechanisms. However, many gaps persist and developing more effective and less risky pain treatments remains a major challenge. Additional challenges exist in translating the mechanistic knowledge into treatments, including regulatory barriers. The IOM report called for better coordination of across NIH institutes and centers by improving study section decision-making on pain proposals, as well as by exploring a range of potential public-private initiatives.

The *Relieving Pain in America* report offered a blueprint for transforming prevention, care, education, and research, with the goal of providing relief for people with pain in America. It offered specific priorities and timelines and called for HHS to develop a subsequent strategy that should be comprehensive in scope, inclusive in its development, expeditious in its implementation, and practical in its application. Most importantly, the strategy was to be far-reaching. That was the charge given to the National Pain Strategy Task Force.

THE NATIONAL PAIN STRATEGY

Following the release of the IOM report, the Assistant Secretary for HHS asked the Interagency Pain Research Coordinating Committee to oversee creation of the NPS. Guided and coordinated by an oversight panel, expert working groups explored 6 important areas of need identified in the IOM recommendations—population research, prevention and care, disparities, service delivery and reimbursement, professional education and training, and public awareness and communication (**Fig. 2**). The working groups comprised 80 experts from a broad array of relevant public and private organizations, including health care providers, insurers, and people with pain and their advocates.

The goal of the NPS task force was to develop a strategic plan to transform pain prevention, care, and education in our country. In contrast to the IOM report, the NPS was to be a tactical report with 3 specific, meaningful, and measureable deliverables from each working group. The draft NPS report was released for public commentary with an expected final release later in 2015. Although the entire report is important, for reasons of space, I will highlight specific sections that are significant for readers of this journal. The information that follows draws from the draft report; the final version may have changes. Much of this information is drawn directly from the NPS report.

Population Research

The IOM report noted that more than 100 million Americans experience chronic pain to some extent. This number encompasses those who have chronic pain of mild impact to those that are highly affected by their pain. It is, therefore, important to differentiate people with high-impact chronic pain from those who sustain normal activities although experiencing chronic pain. To accomplish this goal, the NPS first introduced the term high-impact chronic pain, defined as pain "associated with substantial restriction of participation in work, social, and self-care activities for 6 months or more." This concept of high-impact chronic pain will have significant bearing for those who care for patients with hand conditions because it is those patients who are thought to be the highest utilizers of health care resources.

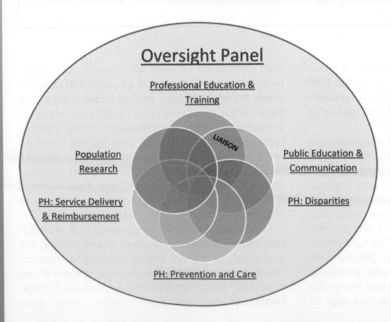

Fig. 2. Structure of the NPS task force including oversight panel and 6 working groups. (*From* National Institutes of Health (NIH). The interagency pain research coordinating committee. National Pain Strategy. Available at: http://iprcc.nih.gov/National_Pain_Strategy/oversight_panel.htm.)

Oversight Panel

Professional Education & Training

LIAISON

Population Research

Public Education & Communication

PH: Service Delivery & Reimbursement

PH: Disparities

PH: Prevention and Care

The challenge will be to identify those patients likely to develop high-impact pain after surgery and to develop preventative measures to reduce this occurrence.

Additionally, the NPS Population Strategy Working Group recommended specific steps to (1) increase the precision of information about chronic pain prevalence overall, for specific types of pain, and in specific population groups; (2) develop the capacity to gather information electronically about pain treatments, their usage, costs, and effectiveness; and (3) enable tracking changes in pain prevalence, impact, and treatment over time, allowing evaluation of population-level interventions and identification of emerging needs.

Prevention and Care

The Prevention and Care Working group noted that greater emphasis needs to be placed on prevention of acute and chronic pain throughout the health care system, environments in which injuries are likely to occur, and those people at increased risk of developing chronic pain. This has particular relevance for clinicians caring for persons with hand conditions. There is a call for more standardized assessment tools and outcome measures through the development of new, rigorously researched approaches. Recommendations are also made to improve pain self-management programs that can help affected individuals improve their knowledge, skills, and confidence to prevent, reduce, and cope with pain.

Disparities

The Disparities Working Group noted that there are groups in which pain is more prevalent, including people with limited access to health care services, racial and ethnic minorities, people with low income or education, and those at increased risk because of where they live or work. The NPS recommends efforts that will increase understanding of the impact of bias and support effective strategies to overcome it, increase access to high-quality pain care for vulnerable population groups, and improve communication between patients and health professionals.

Service Delivery and Reimbursement

Evidence suggests that poor-quality care and higher health care costs are associated with clinical practice variations, inadequate tailoring of pain therapies, and reliance on relatively ineffective and, potentially, high-risk treatments. The Service Delivery and Reimbursement working group recommended a comprehensive biopsychosocial approach to pain care that is grounded in scientific evidence, integrated, multimodal, interdisciplinary, and tailored to individual patient needs. The group noted research and demonstration efforts are needed that build on current knowledge, develop new knowledge, and support further testing and diffusion of model delivery systems.

Professional Education and Training

Strikingly, although pain is a prevalent and common reason for health care visits, most health profession's education programs do not provide adequate pain education. The Professional Education and Training working group noted a need to improve discipline-specific core competencies, including basic knowledge, assessment, effective team-based care, empathy, and cultural competency. Educational program accreditation bodies and professional licensure boards can require pain teaching and clinician learning at the undergraduate and graduate levels. The NPS also recommends development of a Web-based pain education portal that will contain up-to-date, comprehensive, and easily accessed educational materials.

Public Education and Communication

There is a need for greater understanding of important aspects of chronic pain by both members of the public and people with pain. The Public Education and Communication working group recommended a national public awareness campaign involving many relevant public and private partners, including people with pain and their advocates, to address stigma and misperceptions about chronic pain. Additionally, the group recommends a safe-use education campaign targeting people with pain whose care includes prescription medications.

National Pain Strategy Vision

The NPS also set forth the following vision statement, "If the objectives of the National Pain Strategy are achieved, the nation would see a decrease in prevalence across the continuum of pain, from acute, to chronic, to high-impact chronic pain, and across the life span from pediatric through geriatric populations, to end of life, which would reduce the burden of pain for individuals, families, and society as a whole. Americans experiencing pain—across this broad continuum—would have timely access to a care system that meets their biopsychosocial needs and takes into account individual preferences, risks, and social contexts. In other words, they would receive patient-centered care."

Implementation of the NPS will require us to work closely with HHS to advocate leadership from their department. We will need HHS to lead in tasking the relevant stakeholders with implementation of the strategic goals, establishing accountability for progress, and identification and allocation of resources to advance the Strategy. Importantly, this will also require collaboration among healthcare providers, with persons suffering with pain, professional societies and advocacy groups, researchers, employers, payers, elected officials and the media – all on a scale we have not done before. To be successful, we must all be part of the dialogue and the solution, and speak with a single voice. Successful implementation of these strategic goals will create the cultural transformation in pain prevention, care, and education called for in the IOM report and called for by the American public.

FUTURE NEEDS: LEARNING HEALTH SYSTEMS AND PRECISION PAIN MEDICINE

The future of pain assessment, prevention, and treatment will require improvements in clinical education, public and institutional policies and population-level epidemiologic, health services, social science, medical informatics, implementation, basic biomedical, and other relevant research, informed by clinician/scientist interactions. I will focus on an area in which our group is working to advance the recommendations of the IOM report and the NPS.

As noted previously, despite an increase in the number of available pain therapies, more than

100 million people in the United States still live with pain. Little is known about which treatments are best for which patient or even about the efficacy and safety of various treatments over time. In recognizing this conundrum, the IOM report called for "greater development and use of patient outcome registries that can support point-of-care treatment decision making, as well as for aggregation of large numbers of patients to enable assessment of the safety and effectiveness of therapies." Coinciding with this call for patient registries is the recognition that Learning Health Systems (LHSs) are an important aspect of the future of medicine.[6] Learning health systems combine science, informatics, incentives and culture that are then aligned for continuous improvement and innovation The IOM recently extolled the virtues of LHSs,[7] and in 2013 the National Science Foundation convened a workshop where it was declared that LHSs can rapidly inform decisions that have transformative effects on improving health.[8]

The IOM has called for LHSs to use data with advanced analytics to transform care. However, there have been technological barriers to the implementation of LHSs. The Stanford-NIH Collaborative Health Outcomes Information Registry (CHOIR; http://CHOIR.stanford.edu) was developed in response to the IOM Report and the NPS, which emphasized the need to improve the collection and reporting of data on pain (**Fig. 3**). The military has also developed a system to address this need called Pain Assessment Screening Tool and Outcomes Registry (PASTOR).[9] The rest of this discussion will use CHOIR as a model platform. CHOIR is an open

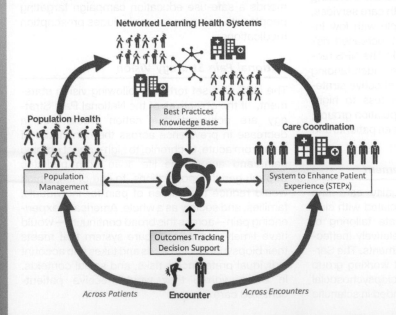

Fig. 3. Open-source public–private partnership learning health system network using Collaborative Health Outcomes Information Registry (CHOIR). (*Courtesy of* Ming-Chih Kao, PhD, MD, Palo Alto, CA.)

Networked Learning Health Systems

Population Health

Best Practices Knowledge Base

Care Coordination

Population Management

System to Enhance Patient Experience (STEPx)

Outcomes Tracking Decision Support

Across Patients   **Encounter**   *Across Encounters*

source, open standard, free, secure, electronic, learning health care system is designed to capture detailed, longitudinal patient-reported outcomes data on physical, psychological, and social health. CHOIR was developed to: inform point of care decision making, provide software based decision making, and act as a platform for (1) comparative effectiveness research, (2) longitudinal outcomes research, and (3) practice based evidence trials.

Although traditional narrowly focused biomedical approaches to medical treatment have been successful for some diseases (eg, infectious diseases), there is a need to efficiently characterize the multidimensional nature of our patients in chronic disease management. Increasingly there is greater awareness in the roles of psychological and social factors in disease incidence, magnitude, and persistence, as well as its associated costs of care. In concert, there are increasingly needs to measure and monitor psychological and social factors in order to better manage these complex diseases. CHOIR integrates NIH Patient Reported Outcomes Measurement Information System (PROMIS) measures to efficiently and rapidly capture 15 to 20 domains of physical, psychological, and social functioning.

The NIH PROMIS measures have been integrated into CHOIR to maximize efficiency in data capture through cloud-based computation with adaptive algorithms for items with wide dynamic range, and computerized adaptive testing. This testing has been shown to reduce patient response burden by as much as 75% and facilitate continued patient participation. An additional strength of PROMIS measures is that they permit for comparisons of individual patients against national population norms.[9,10]

Although evidence-based medicine is the standard for supporting clinical-decision making, the paucity of prospective, placebo-controlled randomized trials in pain medicine has generated an urgent need to accurately and consistently measure relevant patient outcomes with the goal of defining the most safe and effective treatments. There is a need to standardize the assessment and reporting of outcomes to allow for comparison across studies and different patient populations. In addition to prospective, placebo-controlled randomized trials, which can be difficult to generalize due to participant homogeneity, and require a large amount of resources (due to sample size), systematic practice-based evidence may provide more useful data in the form of prospective, observational, cohort studies.[11] Standardized data capture can be included as part of ongoing routine clinical hand and pain management from both patients and providers. CHOIR

was developed to allow for low-cost, large, prospective, observational studies on thousands of patients in a real-world clinic setting. CHOIR, and other LHSs, have the potential to address many fundamental questions regarding pain treatment and efficacy, and will allow for further characterization of optimal patients for specific therapies.[11,12]

In addition to the broad research utility of CHOIR, the system provides computer-assisted documentation, which has proven indispensable and invaluable in delivering comprehensive, targeted interdisciplinary pain treatment. The platform is designed to be customizable to different settings (inpatient and ambulatory), providers, and disease conditions. Use of CHOIR will facilitate real-time comparison of patient data to clinic, national, and disease-specific norms. CHOIR has demonstrated efficiency, low-cost, and minimal burden to staff, providers, and patients, while augmenting clinical care. CHOIR provides rapid real-time, longitudinal feedback to clinicians regarding standardized quantitative outcomes to guide decision-making regarding various treatments.[11]

President Obama has recently called for a Precision Medicine Initiative. Precision medicine is an emerging approach for disease treatment and prevention that takes into account individual variability in genes, environment, and lifestyle for each person. Although President Obama has called for a near-term focus of precision medicine to be cancers, the long-term aim is to apply this knowledge to the whole range of health and disease, including pain management.[13] This effort will require a further advances in molecular biology, –omics (eg, genomics, metabolomics, proteomics), and bioinformatics. Learning health systems will play a significant role in integrating this systems based information to derive accurate prevention and treatment recommendations. These learning health systems and precision pain medicine are within our grasp. Successful implementation will ultimately realize the call by the IOM *Relieving Pain in America* report to provide everyone the best pain assessment, prevention, and treatment.

REFERENCES

1. Institute of Medicine (U.S.) Committee on Advancing Pain Research Care and Education. Relieving pain in America: a blueprint for transforming prevention, care, education, and research. Washington, DC: National Academies Press; 2011. p. 364, xvii.
2. Pizzo PA, Clark NM. Alleviating suffering 101—pain relief in the United States. N Engl J Med 2012;366(3):197–9.

3. Carroll I, Barelka P, Wang CK, et al. A pilot cohort study of the determinants of longitudinal opioid use after surgery. Anesth Analg 2012;115(3):694–702.

4. Carroll I, Hah J, Mackey S, et al. Perioperative interventions to reduce chronic postsurgical pain. J Reconstr Microsurgery 2013;29(4):213–22.

5. Hah JM, Mackey S, Barelka PL, et al. Self-loathing aspects of depression reduce postoperative opioid cessation rate. Pain Med 2014;15(6):954–64.

6. Friedman CP, Wong AK, Blumenthal D. Achieving a nationwide learning health system. Sci Transl Med 2010;2(57):57cm29.

7. Smith M, Saunders R, Stuckhardt L, et al. Best Care at Lower Cost: The Path to Continuously Learning Health Care in America. In: Committee on the Learning Health Care System in America; Institute of Medicine, editors. Washington, DC: National Academies Press; 2013.

8. Friedman C, Rubin J, Brown J, et al. Toward a science of learning systems: a research agenda for the high-functioning learning health system. J Am Med Inform Assoc 2015;22(1):43–50.

9. Cook KF, Buckenmaier C 3rd, Gershon RC. PASTOR/PROMIS (R) pain outcomes system: what does it mean to pain specialists? Pain Manag 2014;4(4):277–83.

10. Gershon RC, Rothrock N, Hanrahan R, et al. The use of PROMIS and assessment center to deliver patient-reported outcome measures in clinical research. J Appl Meas 2010;11(3):304–14.

11. Bruehl S, Apkarian AV, Ballantyne JC, et al. Personalized medicine and opioid analgesic prescribing for chronic pain: opportunities and challenges. J Pain 2013;14(2):103–13.

12. Sturgeon JA, Darnall BD, Kao MC, et al. Physical and psychological correlates of fatigue and physical function: a Collaborative Health Outcomes Information Registry (CHOIR) study. J Pain 2015;16(3):291–298 e1.

13. Collins FS, Varmus H. A new initiative on precision medicine. N Engl J Med 2015;372(9):793–5.

Index

Note: Page numbers of article titles are in **boldface** type.

Hand Clin 32 (2016) 99–101
http://dx.doi.org/10.1016/S0749-0712(15)00143-2
0749-0712/16/$ – see front matter © 2016 Elsevier Inc. All rights reserved.

hand.theclinics.com

Printed and bound by CPI Group (UK) Ltd, Croydon, CR0 4YY

03/10/2024

01040374-0003